FALL PREVENTION BALANCE EXERCISES

FOR SENIORS

——

YOUR 28 DAY PLAN WITH CLEAR ILLUSTRATIONS, SIMPLE EXERCISES & LARGE PRINT TEXT FOR CORE STRENGTH AND STABILITY IN 15-MINUTES A DAY

LINETTE CUNLEY

TABLE OF CONTENTS

CHAPTER 1

INTRODUCTION TO BALANCE

IMPORTANCE FOR SENIORS

As we age, our ability to balance is reduced, and our risk of falling increases. A simple fall might seem harmless, but it can have devastating effects on a person's well-being and quality of life.

Falls have been reported to be a cause of early death and illness for adults over 65 years of age. One-third of older adults living independently in the community will encounter at least one fall per year (Kendrick et al., 2014; Sherrington et al., 2019).

Luckily, balance exercises are one of the tools that can help in reducing the risk of falling and preventing injury.

GOALS AND EXPECTED OUTCOMES

The goal of this book is to teach you practical exercises to enhance your balance, and ultimately help you establish a balance-focused exercise routine to maintain and even improve your daily quality of life.

In Chapter 3, you will assess your balancing abilities with a few simple tests. This will help you to determine which level of balance exercises to begin with.

The balance exercises are presented in Chapter 7, and they are divided into beginner, intermediate, and advanced plans. Each one of these plans is 28 days long, easy to follow, and has clear instructions and illustrations.

At the end of each 28-day plan, you should expect to have an increased sense of balance. You will be able to reassess your balance abilities with the tests from Chapter 3 and take note of your improvements. When you feel ready, you can progress to a more challenging level.

If you successfully follow the 28-day plan, you should feel a greater sense of ease, and gain more confidence in all of the ways you move through your everyday activities.

In the next chapter, we'll review the different types of balance, as well as how balance works. It's important to understand these concepts so you know how to adapt the exercises to your particular needs, and stay motivated as you complete your first 28-day plan.

CHAPTER 2

UNDERSTANDING BALANCE

BASICS OF STATIC AND DYNAMIC BALANCE

There are two types of balance: static and dynamic. **Static balance** is the ability to keep the body in a stable position when the body is not moving. For example, if you're standing in line at the grocery store, you need to be able to keep your static balance with both feet anchored to the floor. You need static balance in order to stand on a crowded bus, sit in a chair with your back unsupported, or hold a kneeling position.

On the other hand, **dynamic balance** is more complex. It is defined as being able to keep a steady posture and alignment even when various body parts are in motion (O'Sullivan et al., 2014, p.187). For example, you need dynamic balance to reach for something that is high up on a shelf, to walk up stairs, or to play pickleball.

Other instances where dynamic balance is important could be turning around unexpectedly, stepping onto a sidewalk, or walking on a busy street.

HOW BALANCE WORKS: VESTIBULAR SYSTEM, VISUAL SYSTEM AND PROPRIOCEPTION

Three systems help us maintain our balance: visual, vestibular, and proprioceptive. Our brain receives information from each of these systems, and then adapts to correct and stabilize our posture. Let's dive deeper into each of these systems.

The **visual system** is composed of our eyes, our optic nerves as well as visual centers in the brain where the visual information will be analyzed. This system allows us to detect movements and determine the position of our different body parts in space. If a part of the visual system is impaired, this could lead to balance issues as it will be more difficult to properly position the body in space.

We can use our understanding of the visual system to modify balance exercises. For example, to make a balance exercise more challenging, we can close our eyes or add movements with our eyes. In contrast, keeping the eyes open during an exercise will typically make it easier to maintain balance.

The **vestibular system** is composed of our inner ear and the vestibular centers in our brain. The main function of this system is to help us maintain balance by detecting and analyzing head movements in space. Inside our ears, we have a complex system that can measure how much our head is turning, tilting, and accelerating. When one of these actions happens, a message is sent to our brain. The information is analyzed, and the brain helps us stay balanced by sending a signal to adjust our posture as needed. When this system is impaired, it can lead to reduced balance as well as symptoms of vertigo, dizziness, and feeling disoriented, to name some examples.

When doing balance exercises, we can use the vestibular system to increase or decrease the challenge. For example, adding head movements can make an exercise more challenging. On the other hand, keeping the head in a static position makes the balance exercise easier.

The **proprioceptive system** is also called the somatosensory system. Essentially, this system helps the body to be oriented in relation to the surface it is standing on. This is possible because the information is transmitted by receptors in our skin, muscles, tendons, and joints. To keep a balanced standing posture, information from the feet, ankles, and hips is especially important (O'Sullivan et al., 2014, p.229). Multiple parts of the body must work together to gather all the necessary information.

There are several ways to challenge the proprioceptive system and increase the difficulty of balance exercises. For example, you can choose to stand on a pillow to make the surface less stable, or choose to not use your hands for support. You can also decrease the difficulty of the balance exercises by performing them on a stable surface, and using your hands to establish more support. The exercise instructions provide options for increasing or decreasing how much you choose to challenge your proprioceptive system.

We can see that balance is complex and requires work from multiple systems at once. When you are at a beginner level, you will start with basic balance exercises that include all three systems. As you become more advanced, you can perform exercises that make each of these systems work harder and challenge your balance further. Working on both static and dynamic balance will be important to make sure that you are ready for all situations that require balance in your everyday life.

In the next chapter, we'll discuss the signs to look out for to notice changes in your sense of balance as well as how to self-assess your current level of balance and choose the most appropriate plan for your needs.

CHAPTER 3

RECOGNIZING AND ASSESSING BALANCE CHALLENGES

SIGNS AND SYMPTOMS OF BALANCE DECLINE

There are many ways to tell if your balance is declining. This chapter will review the common signs and symptoms that indicate you should strengthen your sense of balance. This is not meant to scare you, but simply to make you aware of how to recognize when you start having issues with your balance. The sooner we become aware of these issues, the sooner we can start working toward improving our balance.

Symptoms are what a person feels and signs are what other people can identify for a specific condition, like when a person is experiencing physical imbalance. Here are a few symptoms that the National Institute on Aging suggests you might have a balance problem:

- Fear of falling
- Falling often
- Dizziness or vertigo
- Lightheadedness
- Blurry vision
- Disorientation
- Feeling unsteady when walking

Next, here are some **signs** that a healthcare provider or even a friend or family member might observe if your balance is declining:

- Staggering, shuffling, or dragging your feet
- Swaying when trying to keep a static posture
- Needing to use support when walking
- Trouble changing positions
- Difficulty navigating stairs or sidewalks
- Decreased coordination

COMMON BALANCE ISSUES IN SENIORS

There are many reasons why older adults could experience balance problems. The simple fact of aging is enough to cause balance issues. As we age, our physical and mental capacities decline. This includes diminished muscle strength and coordination of the lower limbs as well as less confidence when walking, and less control over our balance. Combined with decreased mental capacity such as reaction times, this can increase the risk of falling for adults over 65 years of age (Thomas et al., 2019).

Here are some conditions that could affect balance in older adults (National Institute on Aging, n.d.; Saftarie & Kwon, 2018; Peterka, 2018):

- Inner ear problems (vestibular problems)
- Some medications
- Diabetes
- Alcohol consumption
- Heart problems
- Stroke
- Vision problems
- Aging

- Decreased range of motion
- Decreased muscle strength
- Cognitive decline (confusion and memory loss)

As you can see, some causes of balance problems on this list are more serious and will require more than a home exercise program. To ensure you are not missing an important diagnosis, we encourage you to check with your doctor if a significant change has happened in your life recently. If you're unsure if you should undertake a home exercise program for balance your own, please ask your doctor before beginning.

Exercise can improve most common balance problems related to normal aging, loss of range of motion, and reduced strength.

Current research tells us there is a high level of evidence that balance exercises are effective for improving balance and diminishing falls (Sherrington et al., 2019). As mentioned in Chapter 1, the goal of this book is to assist you in your journey to enhance your balance with a 28-day exercise plan.

Simple At-Home Balance Assessment

Now that you understand how balance works, it's time to test your balance abilities.

The following tests will help you decide which of the 28-day plans is the most appropriate place for you to begin. The tests can also be taken again when you complete the plan to see how much you have improved by comparing your results.

Test # 1: 4-Stage Balance Test

Goals:

To test your static balance. To determine your risk of falling. To see how well you can hold four increasingly difficult positions.

How to do it:

- For support, stand near a countertop or a chair that is securely placed against a wall.

- Perform these exercises barefoot.

- Start by holding onto a countertop or the back of a chair, if needed. If possible, once you begin the test try to let go and complete the exercise by balancing on your own.

- You must hold each position for ten seconds to be able to progress to the next one.

- For each exercise, stop if you need assistance or if your feet move from the position.

THE POSITIONS:

Position 1: Stand with your feet close together (they should be touching). Hold for ten seconds. If you were successful, move on to position 2. Otherwise, note how many seconds you were able to hold position 1.

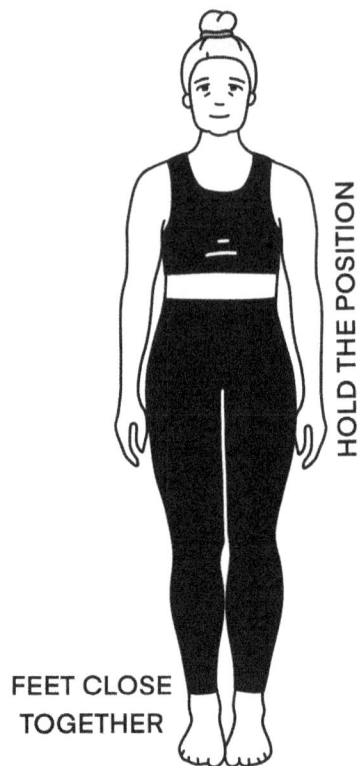

HOLD THE POSITION

FEET CLOSE TOGETHER

Position 2: Stand with your feet in a half tandem position. Pick which foot you want to place in front and make a note of this. The inside of one foot should be touching the big toe of your other foot. Hold for ten seconds. If you were successful, move on to position 3. Otherwise, note how many seconds you were able to hold position 2.

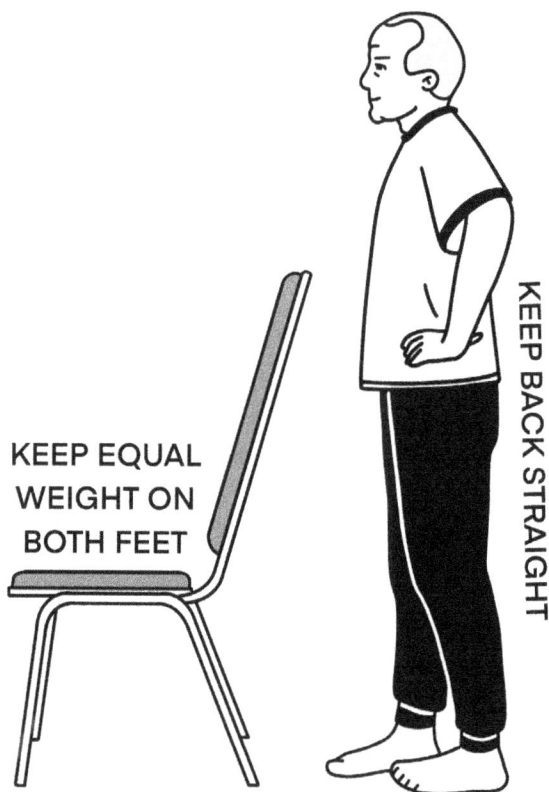

KEEP EQUAL WEIGHT ON BOTH FEET

KEEP BACK STRAIGHT

Position 3: Stand with your feet in a tandem position. Pick which foot you want to place in front and make a note of this. The big toe of your back foot should be touching the heel of your front foot. Hold for ten seconds. If you were successful, move on to position 4. Otherwise, note how many seconds you were able to hold position 3.

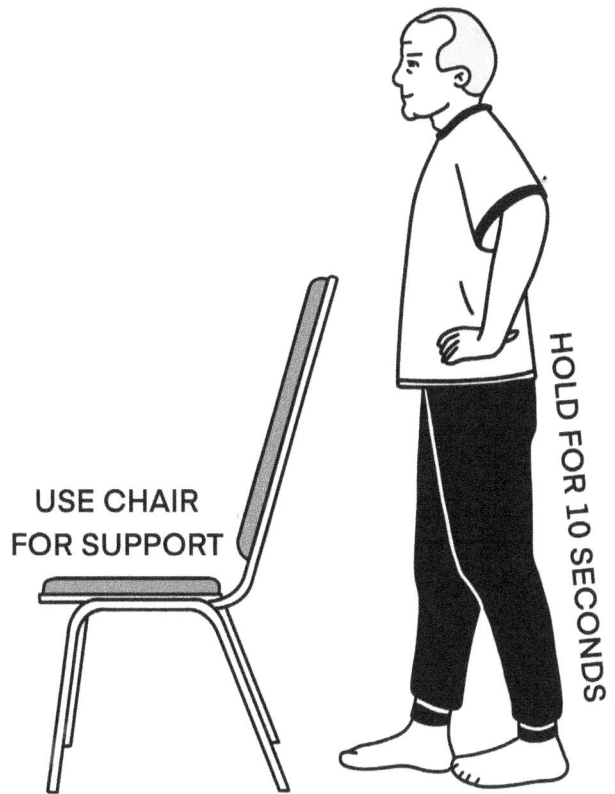

USE CHAIR FOR SUPPORT

HOLD FOR 10 SECONDS

Position 4: Bend one knee and lift your foot behind you, so that you are only standing on one leg. Make a note of which foot you are standing on. Hold for ten seconds.

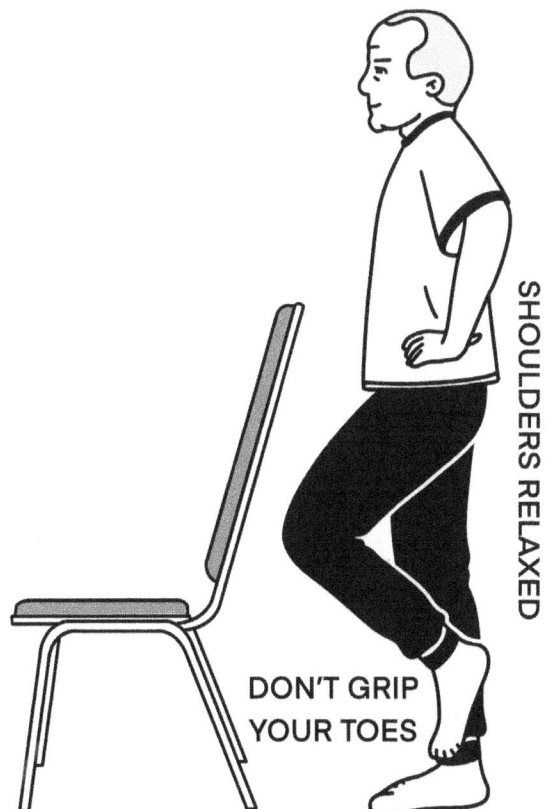

SHOULDERS RELAXED

DON'T GRIP YOUR TOES

If you successfully held each position for ten seconds, you passed the 4-Stage Balance Test with little to no risk of falling. If you didn't quite get ten seconds—don't worry. Use the scoring ranges below to help you assess your current level. Take note of your score so you can compare it when you re-test your balance after you complete your first 28-day plan.

Scoring:

- High risk of falling: you were unable to hold the tandem position for at least ten seconds.

- Medium risk of falling: you were able to hold the tandem position for ten seconds, but you were not able to hold the single-leg stand position.

- Low risk of falling: you were able to hold the single-leg standing position for ten seconds or more.

Test # 2: 30-Second Sit-to-Stand

Goals:

To test your dynamic balance. To determine how many times you can go from sitting to standing in 30 seconds. To determine your risk of falling.

How to do it:

- Place a chair without armrests against a wall.

- The seat of the chair should be about 17 inches (or 43.3 cm) high.

- Sit in the center of the chair with your back upright.

- Your feet should be flat on the ground and hip-distance apart.

- Cross your arms over your chest.

- You can try to stand and sit down a couple of times to test out the movement before you start a timer.

- When you are ready, set a timer with a countdown for thirty seconds.

- Without using your arms, stand up and sit back down as many times as you can in thirty seconds.

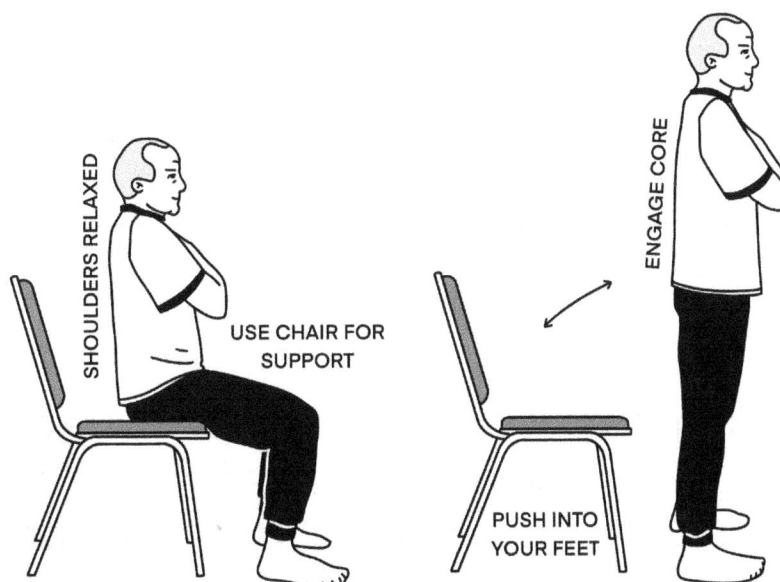

SHOULDERS RELAXED

USE CHAIR FOR SUPPORT

ENGAGE CORE

PUSH INTO YOUR FEET

Scoring:

Note how many repetitions you were able to complete within thirty seconds and use Table 1 below to determine if your score is average, below, or above average. Once you have this information, look under Table 1 to find out what your risk of falling is. This will be important in choosing which 28-day program is appropriate for you.

Table 1:

Normative data according to age and gender for the 30-second sit-to-stand test

Age	Women			Men		
	Below Average	Average	Above Average	Below Average	Average	Above Average
65–69	<11	11–16	>16	<12	12–18	>18
70–74	<10	10–15	>15	<12	12–17	>17
75–79	<10	10–15	>15	<11	11–17	>17
80–84	<9	9–14	>14	<10	10–15	>15
85–89	<8	8–13	>13	<8	8–14	>14
90–94	<4	4–11	>11	<7	7–12	>12

Adapted from "A Health Tool Suite for Mobility Assessment," by P. Madhushri, A. Dzhagaryan, E. Jovanov, & A. Milenković, 2016

- High risk of falling: below average number of repetitions.
- Medium risk of falling: average number of repetitions.
- Low risk of falling: above average number of repetitions.

Test # 3: ABC Scale

The ABC scale is also called the Activities-specific Balance Confidence scale. This one is not a physical self-assessment, but questionnaire that you can fill out.

Go to the last page of the book for instruction on how to download the questionnaire.

Goal: To determine your level of functioning during everyday activities.

How to do it:

- Answer the 16 questions to the best of your ability by giving a score from 0-100% on how confident you are to perform each activity.

- 0 is no confidence in the activity and 100 is maximum confidence.

- If you have never done a specific activity, try to answer by imagining how confident you would be if you had to perform it.

Rate your confidence in performing the following activities on a scale of 0-10.

Scoring:

You will get a score between 0-1600 by adding your score for each question. Take your final score and divide it by 16. The number you get is the percentage that indicates your current level of functioning in everyday activities.

- High level of functioning: a score of greater than 80%
- Moderate level of functioning: a score between 50-80%
- Low level of functioning: a score of less than 50%

Keep the results of your test because you will be able to compare at the end of the 28-day program and see how much more confident you feel during everyday activities.

To summarize, the self-assessment for balance is a crucial part of determining your risk of falling. It is important not to skip the self-assessment. Your score will help you choose the appropriate plan and ensure your safety. It will also allow you to keep track of your progress by retesting yourself after the 28-day plan.

In the next chapter, we'll discuss the benefits of improving balance.

CHAPTER 4

THE IMPACT OF IMPROVING BALANCE

At this point, you should understand how balance works and how to self-assess your balance capabilities. You might now be wondering how improving your balance will help you in your everyday life.

There are many benefits to working on balance that go beyond the simple physical ability of having better balance. Studies have identified the following beneficial effects of balance training (Kendrick et al., 2014; Sherrington et al., 2019; Stanghelle et al., 2020):

- Reduced number of falls
- Reduced number of fall-related injuries
- Reduced fear of falling
- Improved functional mobility

What all these benefits have in common is that they will help you maintain your independence and live a more active daily life.

ENHANCE YOUR INDEPENDENCE

Let's dive deeper into how each balance benefit can help you maintain your independence. First, by working on your balance, you have the potential to reduce the chance of falling. This is great news because falls can have devastating effects. In fact, falls are closely linked to losing confidence, increasing the fear of falling, and having a lower quality of life (Sherrington et al., 2019).

Falling can also lead to injuries that can range from minor to serious. Examples of non-serious injuries could be bruises, muscle strains, ligament sprains, and minor scrapes. More severe injuries could be head trauma, spinal injuries, and bone fractures.

Even if a fall-related injury is not serious, it doesn't mean the problem should be ignored. Other consequences of falling include (Sherrington et al., 2019):

- An increase in healthcare costs
- An increase in pain
- A decrease in mobility and function
- A decrease in daily activities

By working on balance, we can reduce the number of potential falls as well as the injuries that can come with these falls. When you limit your risk of getting injured, you have a better chance of maintaining your mobility and function and therefore preserving your independence.

Finally, the fear of falling brings many consequences. Not only can it affect a person's psychological health, but it can also decrease their mobility and their quality of life (Borowicz et al., 2016).

The more you work on your balance, the more confident you will feel in performing your everyday activities. The skills that you develop while working on balance exercises will transfer into your everyday life. This will allow you to continue doing what you enjoy, and keep your independence for as long as possible.

The key word to remember is independence; this will be your greatest asset. By incorporating balance exercises into your daily routine, you are giving yourself the chance to work toward maintaining or increasing your sense of self-sufficiency and freedom.

In the next chapter, we'll talk about some myths related to aging and activity, and provide some tips to stay motivated with your balance exercises.

CHAPTER 5

OVERCOMING BARRIERS TO BALANCE TRAINING

Harmful assumptions about aging can scare people as they get older and prevent them from living their best life. When it comes to activity and aging, we'll debunk two myths that are important to keep in mind when doing balance exercises.

Myth #1: Elderly people should avoid exercise, and they should take it slow to avoid injuries.

This couldn't be more wrong. It might be difficult to believe that exercise is good for you, or even possible, especially if you are in pain or feel like your body is chronically stiff. On the contrary, if you avoid exercise, you increase the likelihood of experiencing pain and stiffness. In most cases, exercise will make you feel better, and help you keep your independence.

The National Institute on Aging recommends exercise to manage chronic health conditions. They also recommend physical activity to improve physical and mental health. Balance exercises are one of the four recommended types of exercise, along with endurance, strength, and flexibility.

Myth #2: It's too late to learn new things as an older adult.

The second myth that needs to be debunked is that older adults are incapable of learning new things. Not only can you continue to learn new skills as you get older, but you can also improve your performance over time (National Institute on Aging, n.d.).

Additionally, studies show regular exercise positively affects the brain by improving memory skills (Erickson et al., 2011). This is important to remember when it comes to integrating a new skill, like the balance exercises in this book, into your routine. Remind yourself that your exercise routine will positively affect your cognitive and physical well-being.

MOTIVATIONAL TIPS TO START AND STICK WITH BALANCE EXERCISES

When it comes to adding a new regimen to our routine, we know how difficult it can be. In this next session, we'll give you actionable tips to increase your motivation to do balance exercises, and to regularly keep up with your routine.

Here are the recommended tips, with no specific order of importance:

1. HOLD YOURSELF ACCOUNTABLE

In this context, accountability means you hold yourself responsible for completing your balance exercises. One way to do this is to **use a journal or keep a record** of the exercises you complete each day.

In Chapter 7, you will see that each 28-day plan comes with a table where you can take notes and tick the boxes when you have completed the daily exercise routine.

Another way to hold yourself accountable is to **tell a friend or family member** about your plan to complete a balance exercise program. You can ask this person to be your "accountability buddy" by asking them to remind you about your exercises, or to ask you how your exercises are going. You can even ask someone to do the exercise program with you.

2. SCHEDULE YOUR EXERCISE

To be successful in doing your exercises, you need to carve out a dedicated time in your day. **Pick a regularly scheduled time** when you know you will have enough energy to do the exercises. Are you more of a morning person or do you feel like you have a boost of energy right after dinner? Pay attention to what works best for your body. Although you can vary the time at which you do your balance exercises every day, it might be easier to make it a habit if you consistently follow a daily routine.

Another important part of scheduling is to **write it down in your calendar** or **set an alarm** on your phone to remind yourself to do the exercises. This should be non-negotiable, something you do because it has been scheduled. Try to see it as an important appointment with yourself: you can't miss it!

3. SET REALISTIC GOALS

You will feel more motivated if you have a goal to strive towards. The balance goal that you pick will have to be realistic so that you can attain it over the course of the program.

In Chapter 6, we'll guide you through how to set a SMART goal so you can be successful with your balance training.

4. TRACK YOUR PROGRESS

Remember the self-assessments for balance in Chapter 3? Self-assessment is an important part of tracking your progress. By knowing what your baseline is, you can redo the test to see how much you have progressed. This will motivate you to keep going. Try to **self-assess once a month**: you should be able to notice improvement after you complete the 28-day plan.

Another way to track your progress is to **notice how you feel** when performing your everyday activities. The beneficial changes might be subtle at first, but as you progress through the exercise plan, you might notice that you worry less about falling, or that you walk with more confidence and ease. Progress comes in different forms for everyone, so be sure to recognize the subtle signs of transformation in your daily movement.

5. REWARD YOURSELF

Trick your brain into doing the exercises by knowing there is a reward waiting on the other side. This tip is especially useful on days when your motivation is low, and you would rather do anything else. Choose a reward that feels meaningful to you.

For example, you might reward yourself after completing the day's balance exercises with time to watch your favorite show, or enjoy a cup or tea or coffee. You might also choose slightly larger rewards for completing a week of exercises or completing the entire 28-day series, so that you have something to look forward to achieving.

6. CELEBRATE MILESTONES

It is important to celebrate your wins. Studies show that using positive reinforcement when doing exercise can help to keep people motivated (Rivera-Torres et al., 2019).

Positive reinforcement can come from a friend or a family member who sees you doing the exercises and cheers you on or remarks on your improvement.

However, you can also be your own cheerleader. **Journal about your accomplishments**, tell someone how much you have achieved, or just for your effort. Meaningful celebrations might look different for everyone, but whatever your style, make sure to acknowledge it when you have reached a new milestone.

7. MAKE IT FUN

What is something that could make doing 15 minutes of balance exercises more fun for you? Maybe you decide to play some of your favorite music to lift your mood. Maybe you do the exercises in your favorite room of the house. Or, exercise with a friend or family member, to make it a social activity.

What's important is to not take yourself too seriously when doing the balance exercises, and **keep a playful, positive mindset**. If you are getting frustrated because a specific exercise is difficult, remind yourself it will get better with practice.

CHAPTER 6

SAFETY FIRST: PREPARING FOR BALANCE EXERCISES

The most important thing to remember when doing balance exercises is to **always prioritize your safety**. It's important to pay attention to your needs, and always respect your limits.

To help you create a safe exercise environment, follow these crucial steps:

1. **CONSULT YOUR HEALTHCARE PROFESSIONAL BEFORE YOU BEGIN**

   Remember to consult a healthcare professional before beginning a new exercise program, especially if you have high blood pressure, diabetes, or a heart condition. Your provider can let you know what is safe for you.

2. **HOLD YOURSELF ACCOUNTABLE**

   In some of the exercises, you will be asked to hold onto something. When the use of a chair is required, always make sure the chair is propped up against a wall so that it doesn't slide and throw you off balance. Another good option for holding onto a steady surface is to use an empty countertop.

3. **RESPECT YOUR LIMITS**

   Make sure you take the self-assessment before choosing your 28-day plan to ensure you start at the appropriate level. Each exercise in the plan comes with suggestions for how to increase or decrease the challenge, depending on your individual needs. If a specific exercise feels too difficult, don't hesitate to modify it and begin with an easier version.

4. TAKE BREAKS IF NEEDED

Remember to respect your limits. The exercises are designed to be completed in 15 minutes or less per day. However, don't hesitate to rest or take a break when needed. It might take you longer in the beginning, but as you keep going through the 28-day plan, you will build up your endurance.

5. AVOID WEARING SOCKS OR SHOES WITH A SLIPPERY SOLE

We recommend performing the balance exercises with bare feet, as it allows the proprioceptive system to work more efficiently (refer to Chapter 2). However, if you feel uncomfortable doing so or prefer to exercise in shoes, wear a pair that is comfortable and has a non-slip sole.

6. KEEP A PHONE WITHIN REACH, OR WEAR YOUR FALL EMERGENCY DEVICE

This point is important if you live alone. Make sure you keep a phone within reach in case you need emergency assistance during the exercises. If you wear a fall detection device, make sure it's turned on and functional. If you are mindful of respecting your limits, these exercises are designed to be safe and effective. You should feel prepared, so that you can practice the exercises with confidence.

7. STAY HYDRATED

Even though the exercise sessions are only 15 minutes, it's still important to make sure you are hydrated. Drink water as needed before, during, and after your balance exercise session. Being well-hydrated is good for improving your overall health and ensures optimal exercise sessions.

Essential Equipment

The great thing about balance exercises is that they require very little space or equipment to be effective. Most "equipment" needed should be readily available in your home.

Here is a list of equipment we suggest for starting:

- A sturdy chair with a solid base, approximately 17 inches (or 43.3 cm) tall. Do not use a chair with wheels.
- A stopwatch or timer is useful during the self-assessment.
- A space that is quiet and free of clutter.
- A space along a wall that is clear enough to walk ten steps.
- A cushion, if you want to increase the level of difficulty when the exercise provides the option.
- A sturdy step stool approximately 8 or 9 inches tall for advanced level exercises.
- Comfortable non-slip shoes, if you choose to wear shoes.

HOW TO SET A REALISTIC GOAL

In Chapter 5, we talked about ways to improve your motivation. If you set a realistic goal, you will feel more motivated to exercise regularly.

To set a goal for your chosen 28-day balance plan, we suggest using the **SMART criteria** which is a popular framework used across many disciplines for effective goal setting (Doran, 1981).

The SMART acronym stands for:

S=Specific   **M**=Measurable   **A**=Achievable
R=Relevant   **T**=Time-bound

Here is an example of what a SMART goal could look like in the context of a 28-day balance exercise plan:

"I will improve my ability to stand up from a chair by increasing the number of times I can perform the sit-to-stand exercise in the next month. I will do this by following the beginner-level 28-day balance exercise plan."

The goal is specific, time-bound, and relevant: it will help you work on your overall physical health as well as improve your confidence in everyday activities in a measurable way.

Specific: You will improve your ability to stand up from a chair.

Measurable: You can measure improvement using the 30-second sit-to-stand test.

Achievable: You can hit your goal by using the structure of the 28-day plan.

Relevant: Your goal aligns with a valuable plan to improve physical health and confidence in daily activities.

Time-Bound: You set a specific time frame of 28 days to accomplish the goal.

Your SMART goal might be different from this one, but you can still use the SMART structure to make it focused and achievable. As you set your SMART goal, be honest with yourself and consider your current physical condition and what aspect of balance is most important to improve to help you be more independent in your daily life.

You now have all the tools to begin a 28-day balance exercise plan. In the next chapter, we will explain the balance exercises and the 28-day plans according to each level of difficulty.

BONUS CONTENT

We want to see you achieve your goals. To help, I've included bonus resources with you in mind: Easy-to-follow Video Tutorials, Printable Trackers, and Illustrated Posters.

BONUS #1 | **Video Tutorials** - Get unlimited access to easy-to-follow video tutorials that guide you through how to do every exercise in the book.

BONUS #2 | **Printable Trackers and Illustrated Posters** - Stay motivated and track your progress with weekly printable guides.

BONUS #3 | **7-Step Guide to Kicking Fear and Anxiety** - This guide helps you build your confidence and commit to establishing a healthy new exercise routine.

BONUS #4 | **ABC Scale questionnaire** - To determine your level of functioning during everyday activities.

Go to your internet browser and type in **www.getmovefit. com/balance** to register for the unlimited and free portal access. There are no hidden extra costs, this is completely free with the purchase of this book.

The PIN code to unlock your bonus is **on page 111.**

These bonuses are **FREE** and designed to help you achieve your goals.

JOIN OUR COMMUNITY

Did you know that being part of a community that shares your fitness goals can provide a substantial motivational boost?

When you join our community, you'll gain access to knowledge and resources to enhance your journey. Tips, advice, and strategies shared by others who have faced similar challenges can be invaluable.

Join our vibrant and supportive Facebook community to connect with your tribe, navigate challenges, and celebrate your successes.

Go to your internet browser and type in **www.facebook.com/groups/movefitwithlinette/** or within Facebook search **MoveFitwithLinette** to find us.

CHAPTER 7

28-DAY BALANCE IMPROVEMENT PLANS

BEGINNER-LEVEL BALANCE EXERCISES

The beginner-level exercises have been selected to safely and gradually improve your balance.

If you meet the following criteria, the beginner-level exercises are the best place for you to begin:

- You are new to exercise or are returning to exercise after a long break.

- You have a limited range of motion.

- You were at a high risk of falling when you completed your self-assessment for balance in Chapter 3.

- You want to build your confidence by starting with easy exercises first.

All of the following exercises are designed to be simple to learn, and help you improve your balance if practiced regularly. Each exercise includes modifications so that you may adapt the exercise to fit your comfort level.

Following this list, you will find a 28-day plan that gradually integrates each of these exercises. This will help you reach the SMART balance goal that you set in Chapter 6.

SEATED WEIGHT SHIFT (SIDE-TO-SIDE)

- Sit in a chair with an upright posture and relaxed shoulders.

- Keep your back straight; do not rest against the backrest.

- Place your feet hip-distance apart and flat on the floor.

- Rest your hands on your thighs.

- Shift your body to one side to transfer your weight to one buttock, then gently lift your opposite hip.

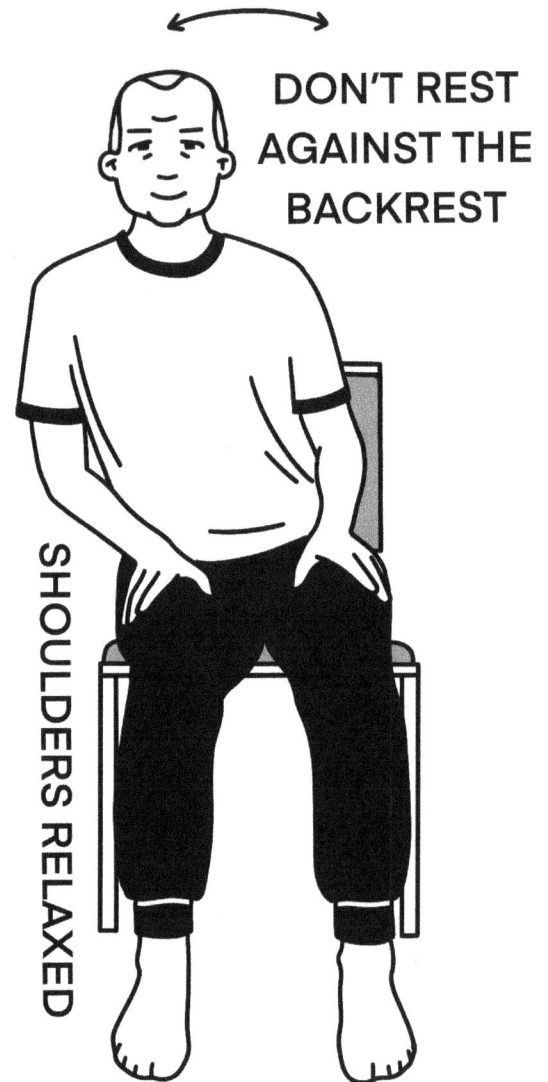

DON'T REST AGAINST THE BACKREST

SHOULDERS RELAXED

BREATHING

Breathe in when you are centered on the seat, and breathe out when you transfer your weight to one side.

MODIFICATIONS

To **increase the challenge**, close your eyes or sit on a pillow. To **decrease the challenge**, support your back against the backrest.

SEATED FORWARD AND BACKWARD PELVIC TILT

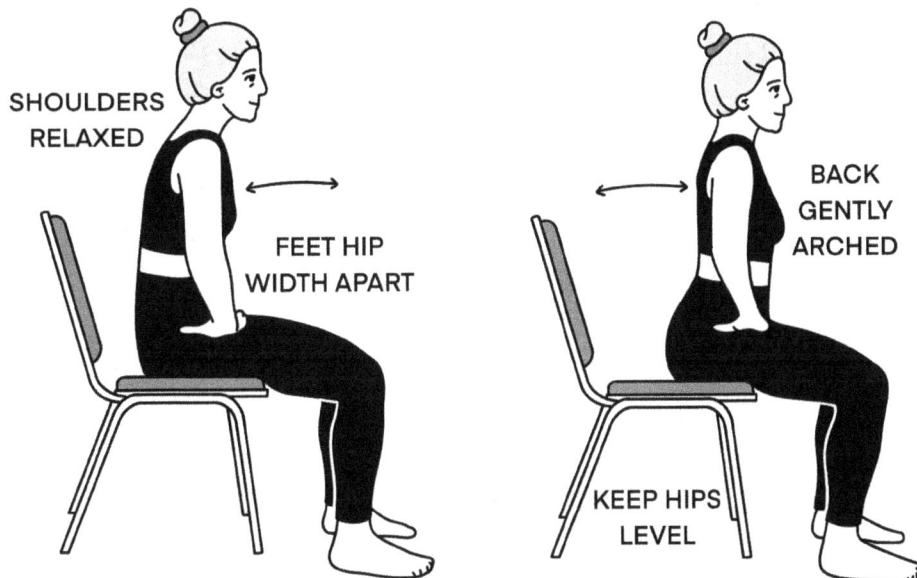

SHOULDERS RELAXED

FEET HIP WIDTH APART

BACK GENTLY ARCHED

KEEP HIPS LEVEL

- Sit in a chair with an upright posture and relaxed shoulders.

- Keep your back straight; do not rest against the backrest.

- Place your feet hip-distance apart and flat on the floor.

- Place your hands on your hips.

- Shift your weight slightly forward allowing your lower back to gently arch (anterior tilt).

- Return to a neutral position.

- Shift your weight backward allowing your lower back to gently round (posterior tilt).

BREATHING

Breathe in when you tilt your pelvis forward, and breathe out when you tilt your pelvis backward.

MODIFICATIONS

To **increase the challenge**, close your eyes or sit on a pillow. To **decrease the challenge**, support your back against the backrest.

SEATED MARCH

- Sit in a chair with an upright posture and relaxed shoulders.

- Keep your back straight; do not rest against the backrest.

- Place your feet hip-distance apart and flat on the floor.

- Cross your hands over your chest.

- Lift your right knee toward your chest, as high as possible without rounding your lower back.

- Lower your right foot back to the floor.

- Repeat the movement with your left knee.

- Alternate both knees to mimic a marching movement.

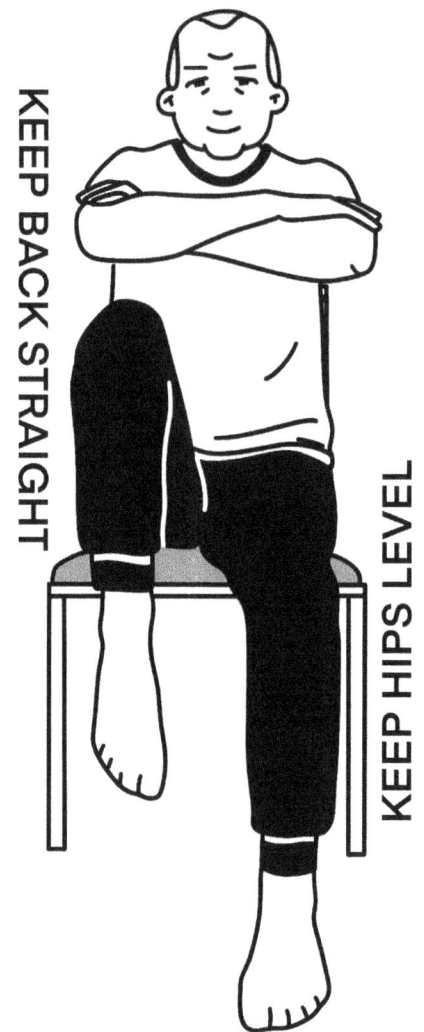

KEEP BACK STRAIGHT

KEEP HIPS LEVEL

BREATHING

Breathe in when you lift your knee toward your chest, and breathe out as you lower your knee.

MODIFICATIONS

To **increase the challenge**, close your eyes or sit on a pillow. To **decrease the challenge**, support your back against the backrest or place your hands on the chair for more support.

STANDING HEEL RAISES (WITH SUPPORT)

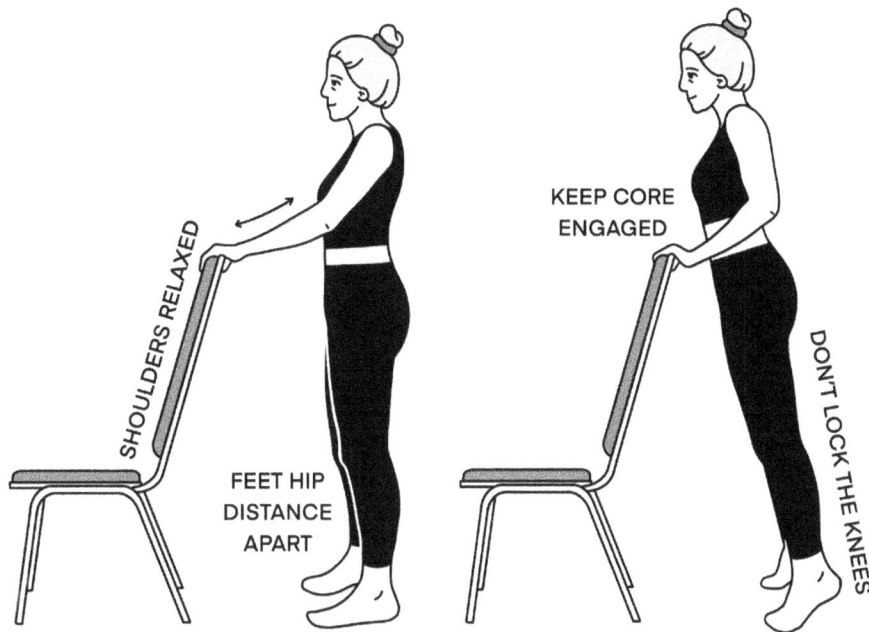

SHOULDERS RELAXED

FEET HIP DISTANCE APART

KEEP CORE ENGAGED

DON'T LOCK THE KNEES

- Place a chair against a wall and stand to face the back of the chair. Hold onto the back of the chair with both hands.

- Place your feet hip-distance apart.

- Keep your back straight and your shoulders relaxed.

- Lift both of your heels off the floor and shift your weight to the balls of your feet.

- Go as high as possible and keep equal weight on both feet.

- Slowly lower your heels back toward the floor.

BREATHING

Breathe in when you lift your heels, and breathe out as you lower your heels.

MODIFICATIONS

To **increase the challenge**, try to release your hold on the chair. To **decrease the challenge**, only lift your heels as high as is comfortable.

STANDING TOE RAISES (WITH SUPPORT)

- Place a chair against a wall and stand to face the back of the chair holding onto it with both hands.

- Place your feet hip-distance apart.

- Keep your back straight and your shoulders relaxed.

- Lift the balls of your feet off the floor and shift your weight to your heels.

- Go as high as possible without falling backward and keep equal weight on both feet.

- Slowly lower the balls of your feet back toward the floor.

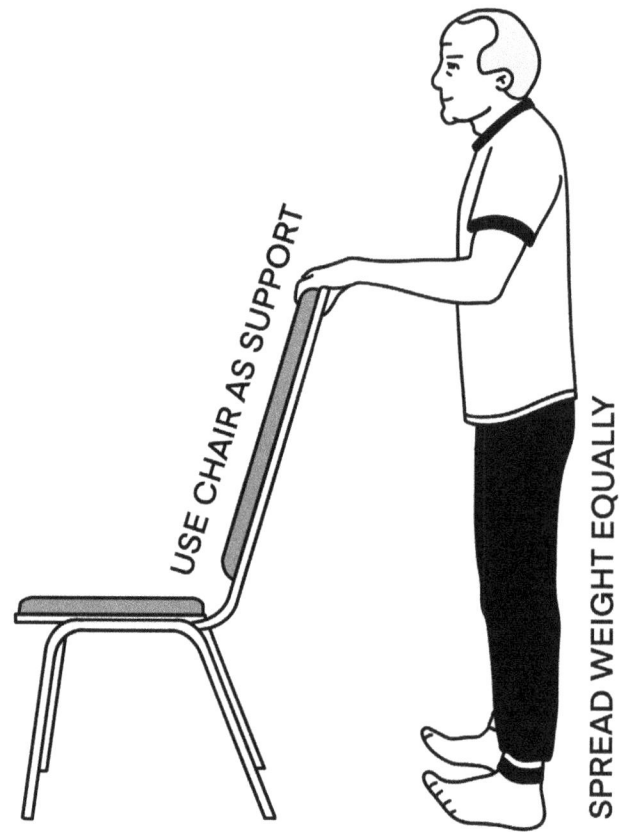

USE CHAIR AS SUPPORT

SPREAD WEIGHT EQUALLY

BREATHING

Breathe in when you shift your weight toward your heels, and breathe out as you lower the balls of your feet back down.

MODIFICATIONS

To **increase the challenge**, try to release your hold on the chair, or alternate lifting the toes one foot at a time. To **decrease the challenge**, only lift the balls of your feet as high as is comfortable.

SMALL KNEE BEND (WITH SUPPORT)

- Place a chair against a wall and stand to face the back of the chair holding onto it with both hands.

- Place your feet hip-distance apart.

- Keep your back straight and your shoulders relaxed.

- Bend your knees and hips as if you were to sit back on a chair.

- Your knees should bend about 20-40 degrees.

- Keep equal weight on both feet.

- Slowly rise back up, extending the knees.

- Keep the entire foot flat on the floor for the duration of the exercise.

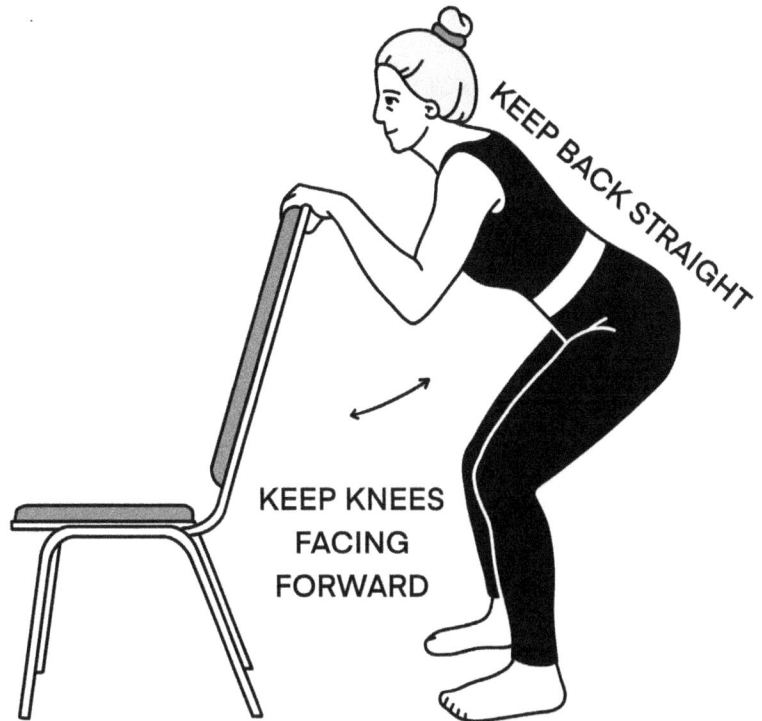

KEEP BACK STRAIGHT

KEEP KNEES FACING FORWARD

BREATHING

Breathe in when you bend your knees, and breathe out as you straighten your knees.

MODIFICATIONS

To **increase the challenge**, try to release your hold on the chair. To **decrease the challenge**, don't go as low when bending your knees.

SEATED FORWARD REACH

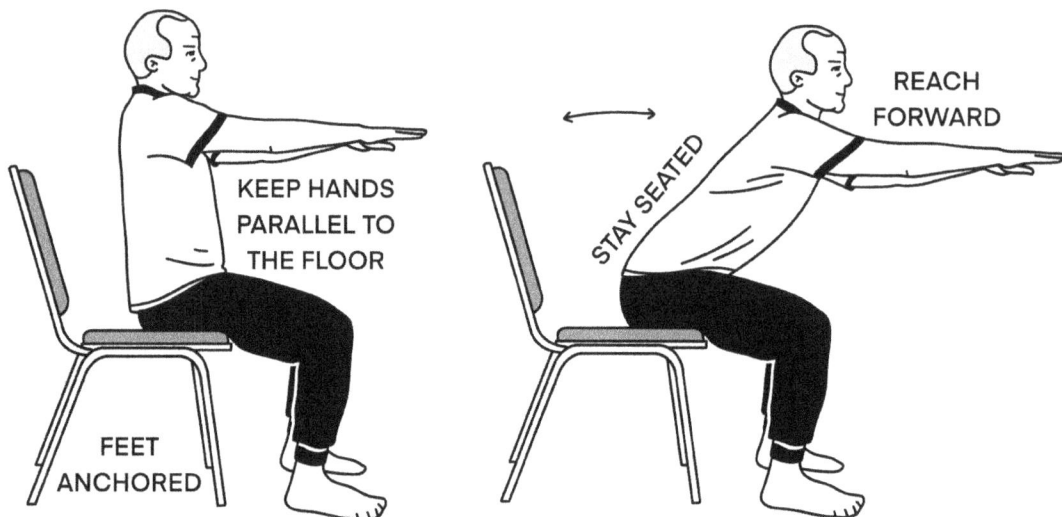

KEEP HANDS PARALLEL TO THE FLOOR

FEET ANCHORED

REACH FORWARD

STAY SEATED

- Sit in a chair with an upright posture and relaxed shoulders.

- Keep your back straight; do not rest against the backrest.

- Place your feet hip-distance apart and flat on the floor.

- Place your hands straight out in front of you with your arms shoulder-width apart at shoulder height.

- Slowly shift your weight forward as if you are reaching for something in front of you.

- Extend as far as you can without falling forward.

- Return to a neutral position.

BREATHING

Breathe in when you are sitting in a neutral upright position, and breathe out as you reach forward.

MODIFICATIONS

To **increase the challenge**, close your eyes or sit on a pillow. To **decrease the challenge**, start with your arms in a lower position (45 degrees instead of shoulder height).

SEATED SIDE BEND

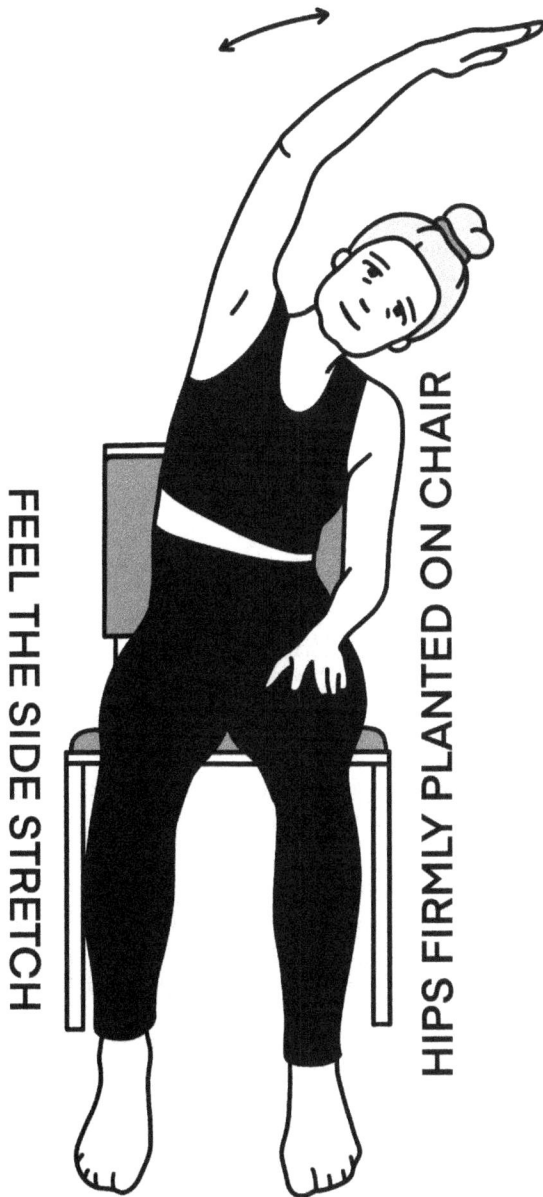

FEEL THE SIDE STRETCH

HIPS FIRMLY PLANTED ON CHAIR

- Sit in a chair with an upright posture and relaxed shoulders.

- Keep your back straight; do not rest against the backrest.

- Place your feet hip-distance apart and flat on the floor.

- Rest one hand on your thigh and reach the other toward the ceiling.

- Begin to reach the raised arm towards the opposite side of your body.

- Control the movement so both buttocks remain firmly on the chair.

- Return to the center and repeat on the other side.

BREATHING

Breathe in at the beginning of the movement to lengthen your spine, and breathe out as you stretch into a side-bend.

MODIFICATIONS

To **increase the challenge**, close your eyes or sit on a pillow. To **decrease the challenge**, modify your range of motion by not bending as far.

SEATED BODY ROTATION

- Sit in a chair with an upright posture and relaxed shoulders.

- Keep your back straight; do not rest against the backrest.

- Place your feet hip-distance apart and flat on the floor.

- Cross your arms over your chest.

- Rotate your torso to one side and try to look over your shoulder.

- Control the movement so both buttocks remain firmly on the chair.

- Slowly come back to the center and repeat on the other side.

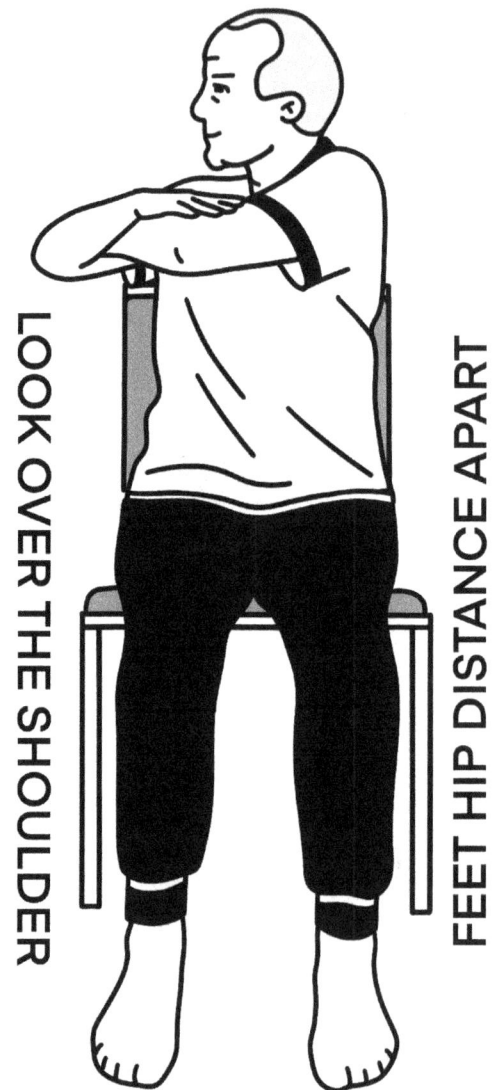

LOOK OVER THE SHOULDER

FEET HIP DISTANCE APART

BREATHING

Breathe in at the beginning of the movement to lengthen your spine, and breathe out as you rotate your torso and neck to one side.

MODIFICATIONS

To **increase the challenge**, close your eyes or sit on a pillow. To **decrease the challenge**, modify your range of motion by not rotating as far.

ASSISTED SIT-TO-STAND (WITH ARMCHAIR)

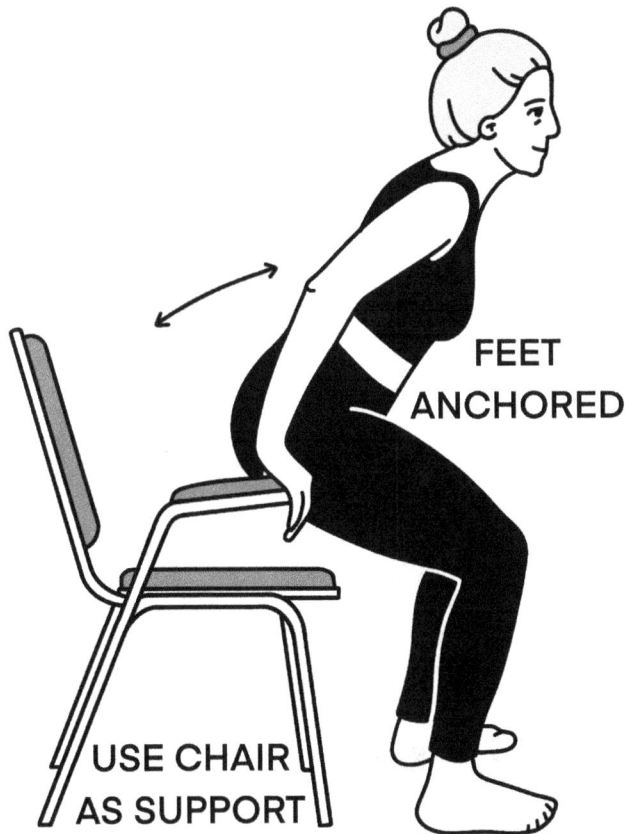

FEET ANCHORED

USE CHAIR AS SUPPORT

- For this exercise, use a chair with armrests.

- Sit in an upright position toward the front of the chair, and relax your shoulders.

- Place your feet hip-distance apart and flat on the floor.

- Rest your hands on the armrests.

- Lean your torso forward as you push into the armrests with your hands, and rise up into a standing position.

- Maintain control as you reverse the motion and sit back down.

BREATHING

Breathe in at the beginning of the movement to lengthen your spine, and breathe out as you move from sitting to standing. Breathe in as you sit back down.

MODIFICATIONS

To **increase the challenge**, use only one armrest. To **decrease the challenge**, place books or a cushion under your buttocks so you have less range of motion to cover.

SINGLE-LEG HEEL RAISES (WITH SUPPORT)

- Place a chair against a wall and stand facing the back of the chair while holding onto it with both hands.

- Place your feet hip-distance apart.

- Keep your back straight and your shoulders relaxed.

- Bend one knee slightly, so that you are only standing on one leg.

- Keep your hips level and your thighs parallel.

- Shift your weight to the ball of the foot you are standing on, and lift the heel of the same foot as high as possible. Be sure to keep your knees straight but not locked.

- Slowly lower your heel back toward the floor.

- Repeat this movement on both sides.

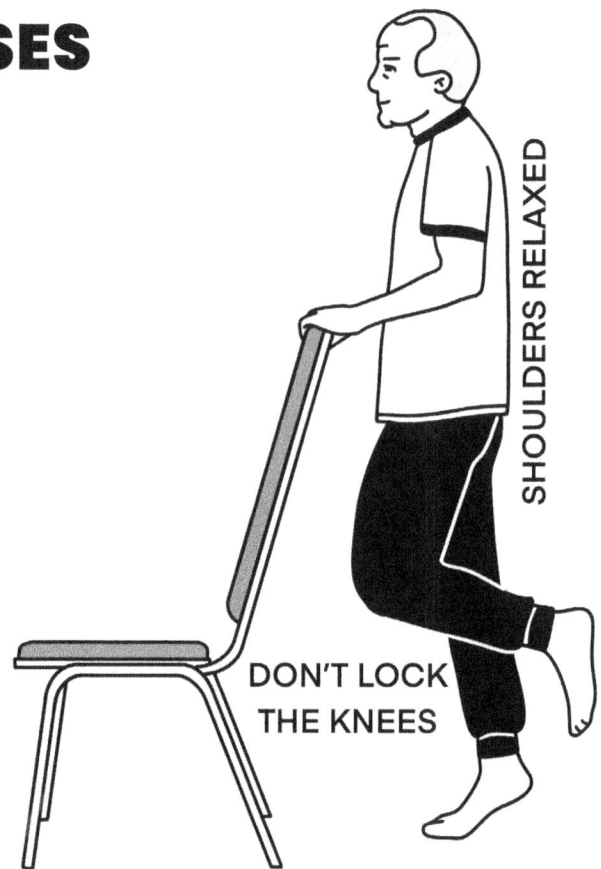

SHOULDERS RELAXED

DON'T LOCK THE KNEES

BREATHING

Breathe in when you lift your heel, and breathe out as you lower your heel.

MODIFICATIONS

To **increase the challenge**, try to release your hold on the chair. To **decrease the challenge**, moderate how high you lift your heel, or do exercise with two feet on the floor.

ROCKING BACK AND FORTH (WITH SUPPORT)

- Place a chair against a wall and stand facing the back of the chair while holding onto it with both hands.

- Place your feet hip-distance apart with equal weight on both feet.

- Keep your back straight and your shoulders relaxed.

- Begin to slowly rock backward to shift your weight in your heels. Your toes should lift from the floor.

- Make your way back to the center and rock forward to shift the weight to the balls of your feet. Your heels should lift off the floor.

- Rock back and forth, controlling both directions of the movement.

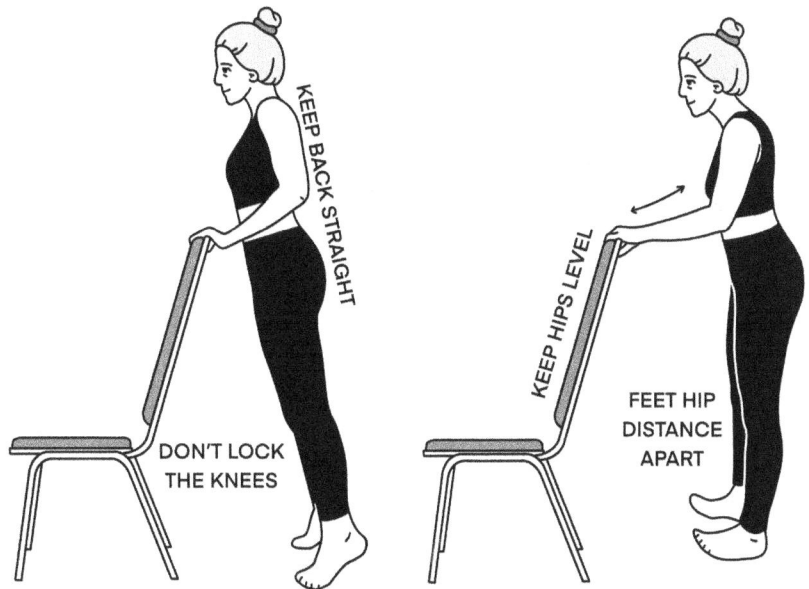

KEEP BACK STRAIGHT

DON'T LOCK THE KNEES

KEEP HIPS LEVEL

FEET HIP DISTANCE APART

BREATHING

Maintain steady breathing throughout the whole exercise.

MODIFICATIONS

To **increase the challenge**, try to release your hold on the chair. To **decrease the challenge**, don't go as far backward or forward when you shift your weight.

TANDEM STANCE (WITH SUPPORT)

- Place a chair against a wall and stand facing the back of the chair while holding onto it with both hands.

- Place your feet in a tandem stance with the heel of one foot directly in front of the toes of the other foot.

- Keep your back straight and your shoulders relaxed.

- Maintain your balance with an equal amount of weight on both feet.

- Do not grip your toes.

- Repeat this exercise by alternating which foot is placed in front of the other.

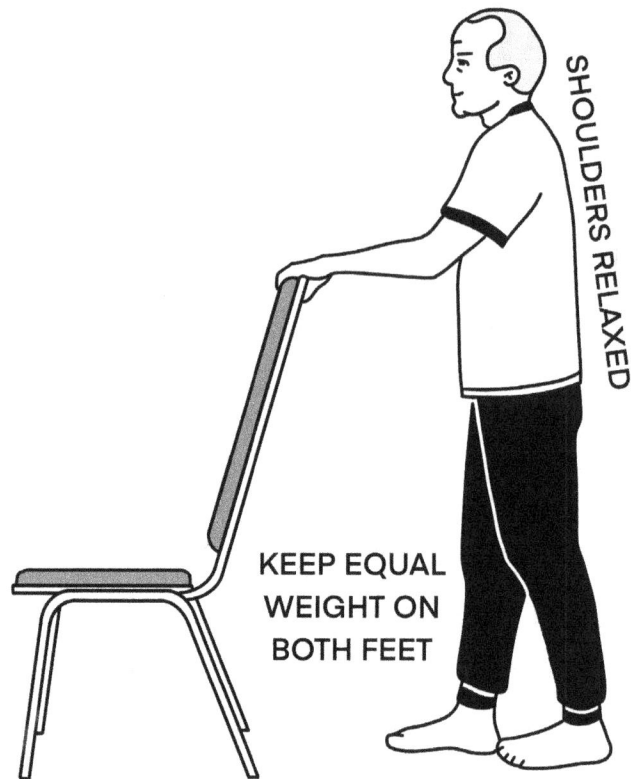

SHOULDERS RELAXED

KEEP EQUAL WEIGHT ON BOTH FEET

BREATHING

Maintain steady breathing throughout the whole exercise.

MODIFICATIONS

To **increase the challenge**, try to release your hold on the chair. To **decrease the challenge**, widen your stance and keep your feet in a staggered position so that one isn't lined up directly behind the other, but a little bit to the side.

NARROW STANCE (WITHOUT SUPPORT)

- Place a chair against a wall and stand facing the back of the chair while holding onto it with both hands.

- Place your feet side by side so they are touching each other.

- Keep your back straight and your shoulders relaxed.

- Let go of the chair and place your hands on your hips.

- Maintain your balance with an equal amount of weight on both feet.

- Do not grip your toes.

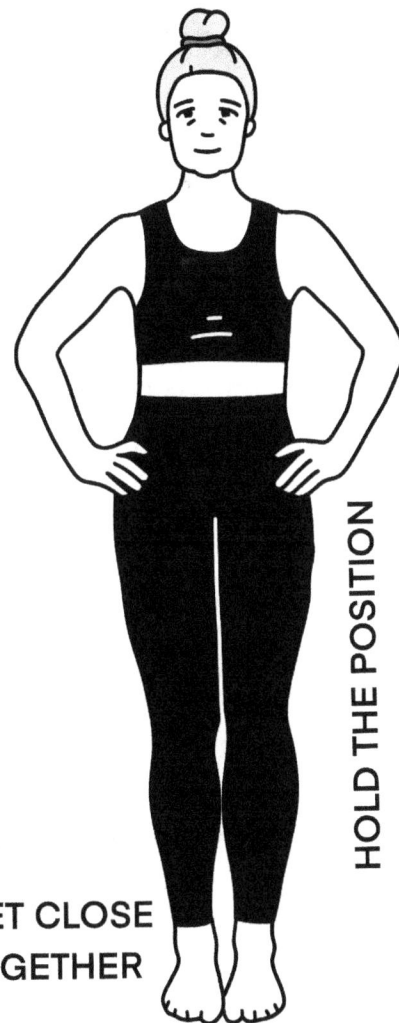

HOLD THE POSITION

FEET CLOSE TOGETHER

BREATHING

Maintain steady breathing throughout the whole exercise.

MODIFICATIONS

To **increase the challenge**, try to release your hold on the chair. To **decrease the challenge**, widen the space between your feet so it becomes easier, but remains challenging.

STANDING WITH A SIDE-TO-SIDE WEIGHT SHIFT

- Place a chair against a wall and stand facing the back of the chair while holding onto it with both hands.

- Place your feet hip-distance apart.

- Keep your back straight and your shoulders relaxed.

- Let go of the chair and place your hands on your hips.

- Maintain an equal amount of weight on both feet.

- Slowly shift your weight to one side to transfer your weight to one foot while lightly touching the floor with your other foot.

- Come back to the center.

- Shift your weight to the other side in the same way.

- Do not grip your toes.

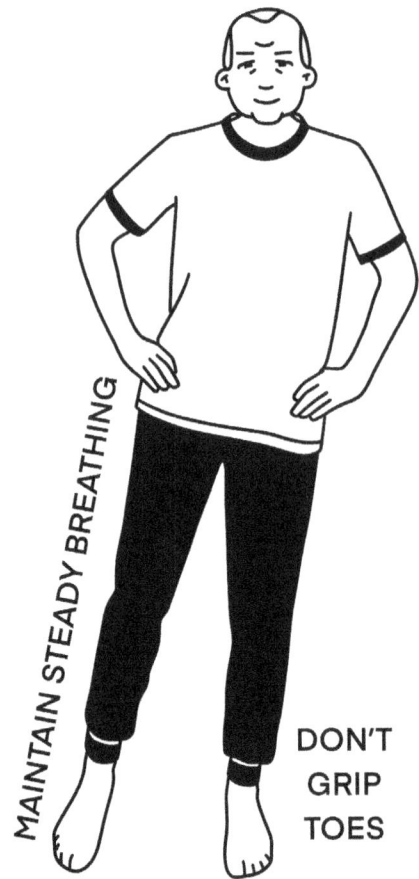

MAINTAIN STEADY BREATHING

DON'T GRIP TOES

BREATHING

Maintain steady breathing throughout the whole exercise.

MODIFICATIONS

To **increase the challenge**, narrow your base of support so that your feet are touching each other. To **decrease the challenge**, hold on to the back of the chair.

SINGLE-LEG STAND (WITH SUPPORT)

- Place a chair against a wall and stand facing the back of the chair while holding onto it with both hands.

- Stand with your feet hip-distance apart.

- Keep your back straight and your shoulders relaxed.

- Bend one knee and lift your foot behind you, so that you are only standing on one leg.

- Maintain your balance with the weight evenly distributed on the four corners of your foot.

- Do not grip your toes.

- Repeat this exercise with your other foot.

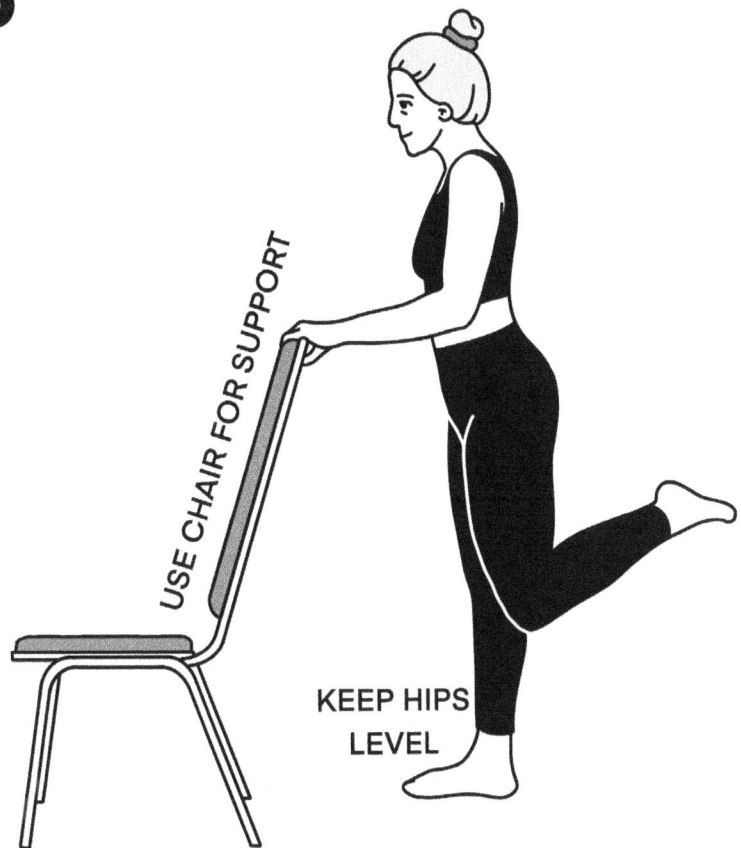

USE CHAIR FOR SUPPORT

KEEP HIPS LEVEL

BREATHING

Maintain steady breathing throughout the whole exercise.

MODIFICATIONS

To **increase the challenge**, try to release your hold on the chair. To **decrease the challenge**, lightly rest the toes of your raised foot on the floor.

28-DAY BEGINNER-LEVEL BALANCE PLAN

Now that you have read through the beginner-level exercises for balance, try to integrate these exercises into the following 28-day plan. Use the following tables to keep yourself accountable and track your progress each week.

The plan is divided into **four weeks**; each week will get progressively more challenging. Please refer to the images and instructions to safely and correctly perform each exercise.

Each week, you will perform **six exercises**. We recommend doing these **five or six times per week**. Include at least one rest day every week. If you follow the recommended number of repetitions, it should take 15 minutes or less to complete these balance exercises every day.

In addition to the exercises, we also recommend **walking for 30 minutes, at least five times per week**. You can divide your walking into separate sessions if you prefer doing so.

For example, you could walk three times a day for 10 minutes, or two times a day for 15 minutes. Remember that every exercise session you can complete is beneficial.

Feel free to modify the recommended walking routine to best fit your individual needs. You can walk without any assistance if you can do so safely, or use an assisted device such as a cane or a walker if needed. What is most important is that you stay safe and work within your limits.

BEGINNER–LEVEL BALANCE EXERCISES

WEEK 1

EXERCISE	REPETITIONS	DAY						
		MON	TUE	WED	THU	FRI	SAT	SUN
Seated weight shift (side-to-side)	10 reps (x2)							
Seated forward / backward pelvic tilt	10 reps (x2)							
Seated march	10 reps (x2)							
Standing heel raises (with support)	15 reps (x2)							
Standing toe raises (with support)	15 reps (x2)							
Small knee bend (with support)	15 reps (x2)							
Walking	30 minutes							

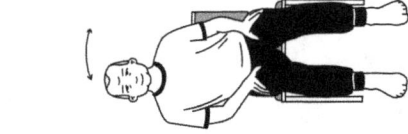

Seated weight shift (side-to-side)

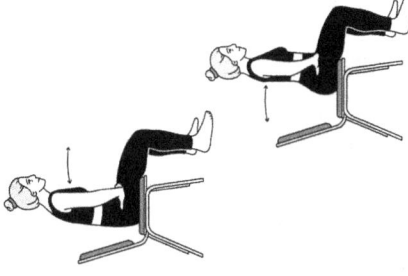

Seated forward / backward pelvic tilt

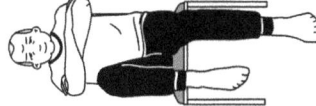

Seated march

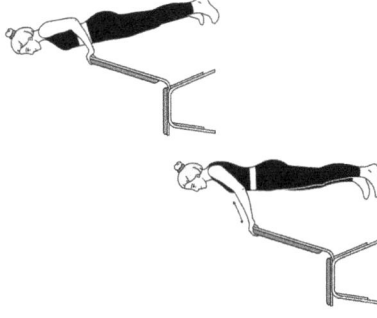

Standing heel raises (with support)

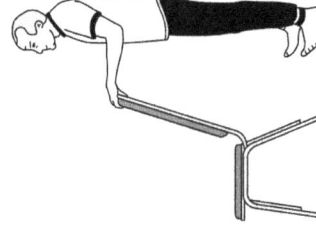

Standing toe raises (with support)

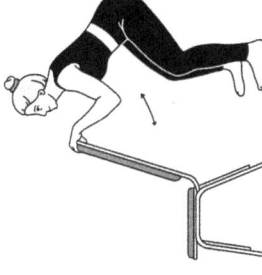

Small knee bend (with support)

BEGINNER–LEVEL BALANCE EXERCISES

WEEK 2

EXERCISE	REPETITIONS	MON	TUE	WED	THU	FRI	SAT	SUN
				DAY				
Seated forward reach	10 reps (x2)							
Seated side bend	10 reps (x2)							
Seated body rotation	10 reps (x2)							
Standing heel raises (with support) Challenge: Perform with less support	15 reps (x2)							
Standing toe raises (with support)	20 reps (x2)							
Small knee bend (with support) Challenge: Perform with less support	15 reps (x2)							
Walking	30 minutes							

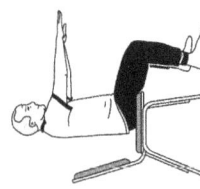

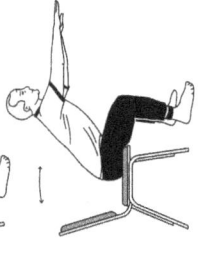

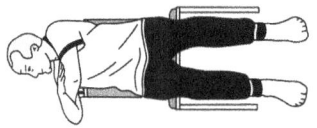

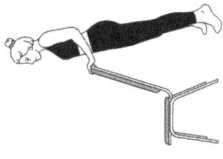

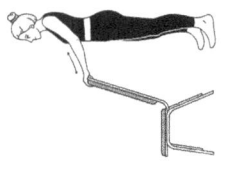

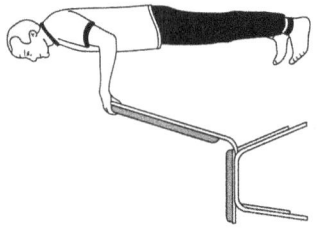

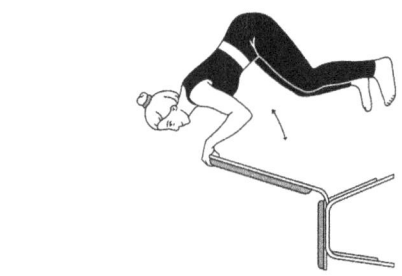

Seated forward reach

Seated side bend

Seated body rotation

Standing heel raises (with support)

Standing toe raises (with support)

Standing toe raises (with support)

Small knee bend (with support)

BEGINNER–LEVEL BALANCE EXERCISES

EXERCISE	REPETITIONS	DAY						
		MON	TUE	WED	THU	FRI	SAT	SUN
Assisted sit–to–stand (with armchair)	10 reps (x2)							
Single–leg heel raises (with support)	10 reps (x2)							
Rocking back and forth (with support)	10 reps (x2)							
Small knee bend (with support) Challenge: Perform without support	10 reps (x2)							
Tandem stance (with support) Challenge: Perform without support	Hold for 10 (x3)							
Narrow stance (without support)	Hold for 10 (x3)							
Walking	30 minutes							

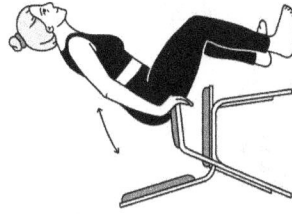

Assisted sit–to–stand (with armchair)

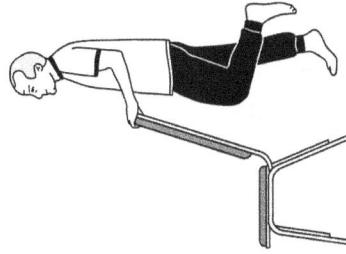

Single–leg heel raises (with support)

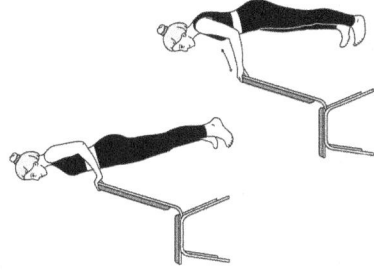

Rocking back and forth (with support)

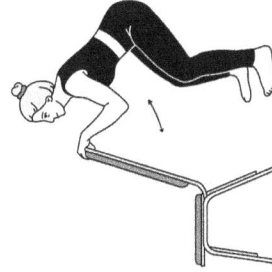

Small knee bend (with support)

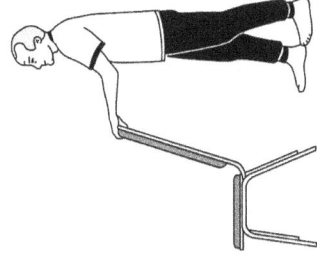

Tandem stance (with support)

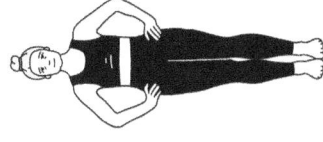

Narrow stance (without support)

BEGINNER-LEVEL BALANCE EXERCISES

EXERCISE	REPETITIONS	DAY						
		MON	TUE	WED	THU	FRI	SAT	SUN
Assisted sit-to-stand (with armchair) Challenge: Perform without support	10 reps (x2)							
Single-leg heel raises (with support)	10 reps (x2)							
Rocking back and forth (with support) Challenge: Perform without support	10 reps (x2)							
Tandem stance (with support) Challenge: Perform without support	Hold for 10 (x3)							
Standing with a side-to-side weight shift	10 reps (x2)							
Single-leg stand (with support)	Hold for 10 (x3)							
Walking	30 minutes							

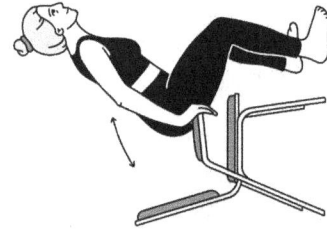

Assisted sit-to-stand (with armchair)

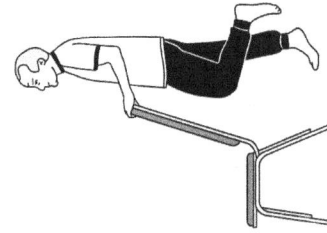

Single-leg heel raises (with support)

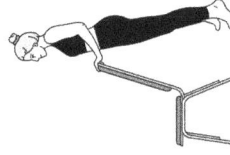

Rocking back and forth (with support)

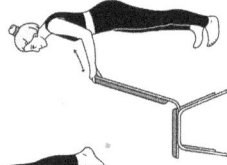

Tandem stance (with support)

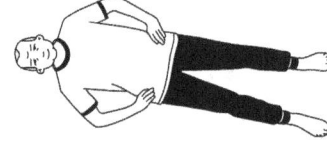

Standing with a side-to-side weight shift

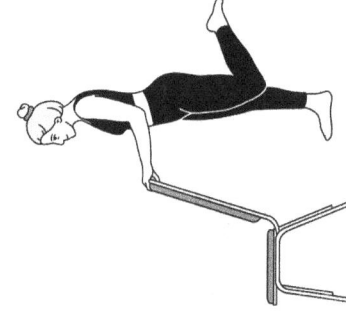

Single-leg stand (with support)

INTERMEDIATE-LEVEL BALANCE EXERCISES

The intermediate-level exercises have been selected to further challenge your balance and improve your coordination.

These exercises include more challenging movements than those at the beginner-level.

If you meet the following criteria, you are ready for the intermediate-level exercises:

- You have completed the beginner-level program and are ready for a new challenge.

- You were at (or below) a **medium risk of falling** when you completed your self-assessment for balance in Chapter 3.

The following exercises are designed to be simple to learn, and help you challenge and improve your balance if practiced regularly. Each exercise includes modifications so that you may adapt the exercise to fit your comfort level.

Some of these exercises will suggest you use a prop like a cushion to challenge your balance. Please remember that it's always optional and isn't a requirement if you don't feel comfortable doing so. Following the list of intermediate exercises, you will find a 28-day plan that gradually integrates each of these exercises. This will help you reach the SMART balance goal that you have set in Chapter 6.

UNASSISTED SIT-TO-STAND

- For this exercise, refrain from using armrests, if your chair has them.

- Sit in an upright position toward the front of the chair and relax your shoulders.

- Place your feet hip-distance apart and flat on the floor.

- Extend your arms out in front of you at shoulder height.

- Lean your torso forward as you push into your feet and rise into a standing position.

- Maintain control as you reverse the motion and sit back down.

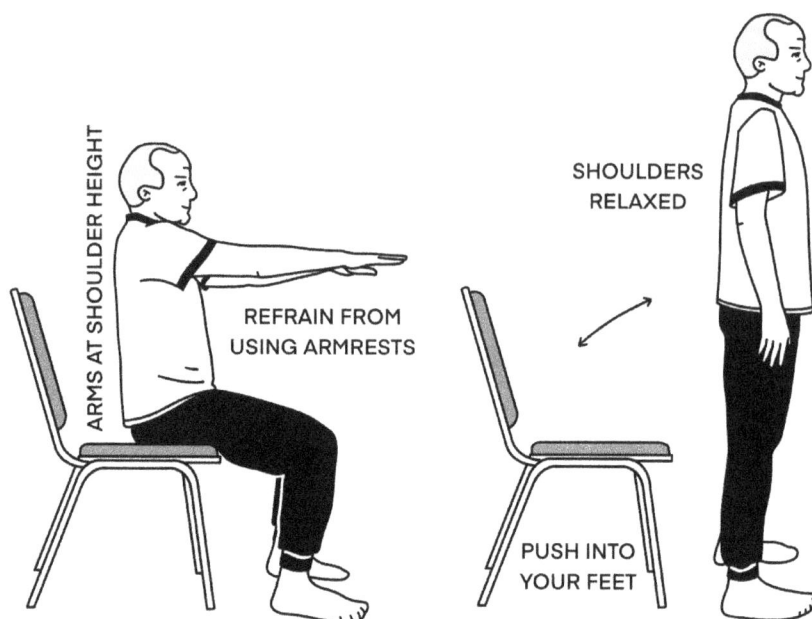

ARMS AT SHOULDER HEIGHT

REFRAIN FROM USING ARMRESTS

SHOULDERS RELAXED

PUSH INTO YOUR FEET

BREATHING

Breathe in at the beginning of the movement to lengthen your spine, and breathe out as you move from sitting to standing. Breathe in as you sit back down.

MODIFICATIONS

To **increase the challenge**, cross your arms over your chest or use a lower chair. To **decrease the challenge**, place books or a cushion under your buttocks so you have less range of motion to cover.

SINGLE-LEG HEEL RAISES (WITH LIGHT SUPPORT)

- Place a chair against a wall and stand facing the back of the chair; lightly rest your hands on the back of the chair to steady yourself.

- Place your feet hip-distance apart.

- Keep your back straight and your shoulders relaxed.

- Bend one knee and lift your foot behind you, so that you are only standing on one leg.

- Keep your hips level and your thighs parallel.

- Shift your weight to the ball of the foot you are standing on, and lift the heel of the same foot as high as possible. Be sure to keep your knees straight but not locked.

- Slowly lower your heel back toward the floor.

- Repeat this movement on both sides.

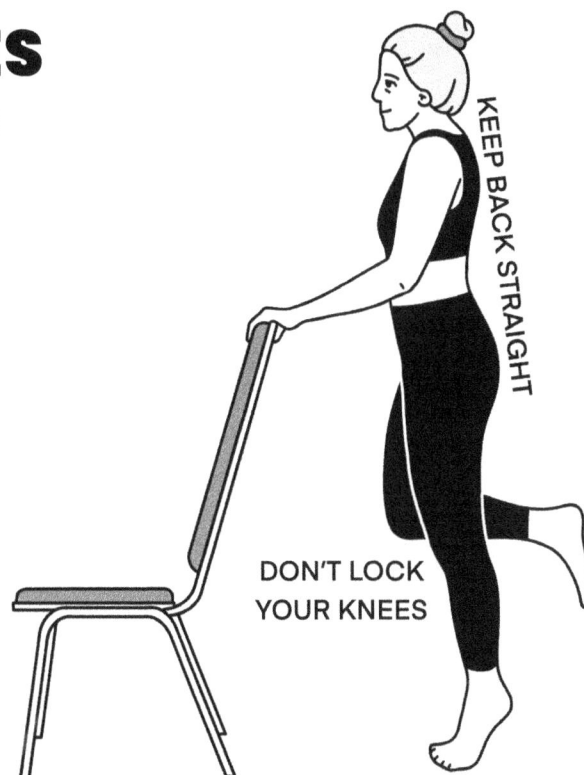

KEEP BACK STRAIGHT

DON'T LOCK YOUR KNEES

BREATHING

Breathe in when you lift your heel, and breathe out as you lower your heel.

MODIFICATIONS

To **increase the challenge**, try to release your hold on the chair. To **decrease the challenge**, moderate how high you lift your heel, or put more weight into your fingers to support you.

SIDE LEG RAISES (WITH SUPPORT)

- Place a chair against a wall and stand so that one of your hips is near the back of the chair.

- Hold onto the chair with your nearest hand for support. For example, you want to hold on to the chair with your right hand if the leg left is the one that will be lifting first out to the side.

- Place your feet hip-distance apart.

- Keep your back straight and your shoulders relaxed.

- Lift the leg that is farthest from the chair out to the side as far as you comfortably can without rotating the pelvis or side-bending your trunk.

- Keep your spine tall.

- Slowly lower your leg back toward your standing leg.

- Repeat this movement on both sides.

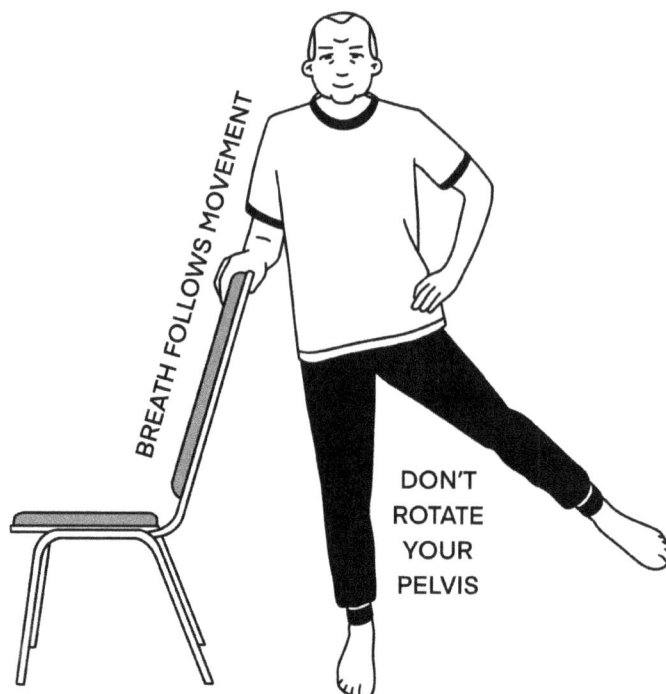

BREATH FOLLOWS MOVEMENT

DON'T ROTATE YOUR PELVIS

BREATHING

Breathe in when you lift your leg, and breathe out as you lower your leg.

MODIFICATIONS

To **increase the challenge**, try to release your hold on the chair, or place both hands on your hips. To **decrease the challenge**, face the back of the chair and hold onto it with both hands or decrease the range of motion when you lift your leg.

TANDEM STANCE (WITHOUT SUPPORT)

- Place a chair against a wall and stand facing the back of the chair while holding onto it with both hands.

- Place your feet in a tandem stance with the heel of one foot directly in front of the toes of the other foot.

- Let go of the chair and place your hands on your hips.

- Try not to use your hands if possible, but steady yourself on the back of the chair if needed.

- Keep your back straight and your shoulders relaxed.

- Maintain your balance with an equal amount of weight on both feet.

- Do not grip your toes.

- Repeat this exercise by alternating which foot is placed in front of the other.

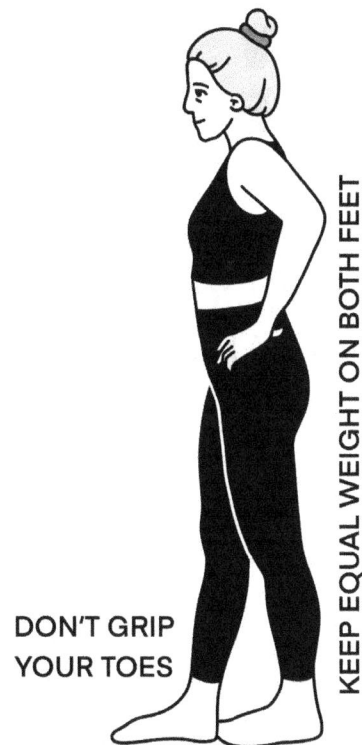

KEEP EQUAL WEIGHT ON BOTH FEET

DON'T GRIP YOUR TOES

BREATHING

Maintain steady breathing throughout the whole exercise.

MODIFICATIONS

To **increase the challenge**, stand on a cushion. To **decrease the challenge**, widen your stance and keep your feet in a staggered position so that one isn't lined up directly behind the other, but a little bit to the side.

NARROW STANCE (WITH NECK ROTATION)

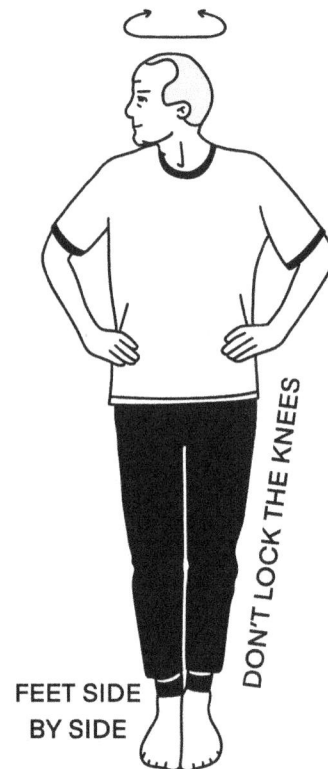

FEET SIDE BY SIDE

DON'T LOCK THE KNEES

- Place a chair against a wall and stand facing the back of the chair while holding onto it with both hands.

- Place your feet side by side so they are touching each other.

- Keep your back straight and your shoulders relaxed.

- Let go of the chair and place your hands on your hips.

- Start turning your head to look to the left, come back through the center, and turn your head to the right.

- Maintain your balance with an equal amount of weight on both feet.

- Do not grip your toes.

BREATHING

Maintain steady breathing throughout the whole exercise.

MODIFICATIONS

To **increase the challenge**, stand on a cushion, or instead of the neck rotations, you can close your eyes. To **decrease the challenge**, widen the space between your feet to provide more balance, or eliminate the neck rotations.

SINGLE-LEG STAND (WITHOUT SUPPORT)

- Place a chair against a wall and stand facing the back of the chair while holding onto it with both hands.

- Stand with your feet hip-distance apart.

- Keep your back straight and your shoulders relaxed.

- Bend one knee and lift your foot behind you, so that you are only standing on one leg.

- Let go of the chair and place your hands on your hips.

- Maintain your balance with the weight evenly distributed on the four corners of your standing foot.

- Do not grip your toes.

- Repeat this exercise with your other foot.

- Try not to use your hands if possible, but steady yourself on the back of the chair if needed.

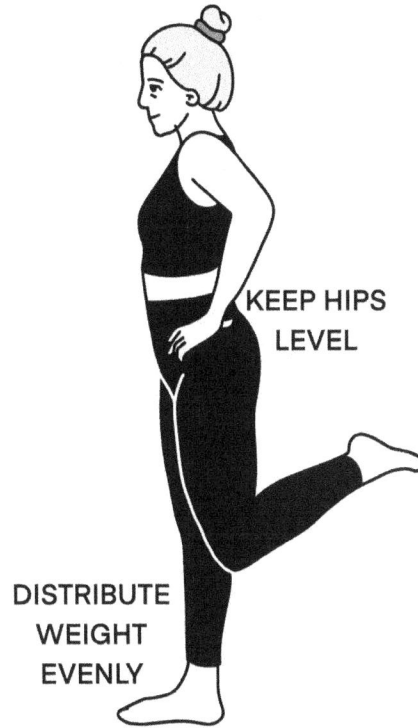

KEEP HIPS LEVEL

DISTRIBUTE WEIGHT EVENLY

BREATHING

Maintain steady breathing throughout the whole exercise.

MODIFICATIONS

To **increase the challenge**, stand on a cushion or close your eyes. To **decrease the challenge**, lightly rest the toes of your raised foot on the floor or rest the fingers of one hand on the back of the chair for additional support.

TOE WALKING

- Stand next to a wall with enough space to walk forward without any obstacles.

- Facing away from the wall, put one hand on the wall for support.

- Place your feet hip-distance apart.

- Keep your back straight and your shoulders relaxed.

- Shift your weight to the balls of both feet and lift the heels as high as possible. Be sure to keep your knees straight but not locked.

- Begin to walk forward keeping the heels lifted.

- Look forward as you walk; do not look down at your feet.

- Relax your heels down after ten steps, turn around, and repeat by walking in the other direction.

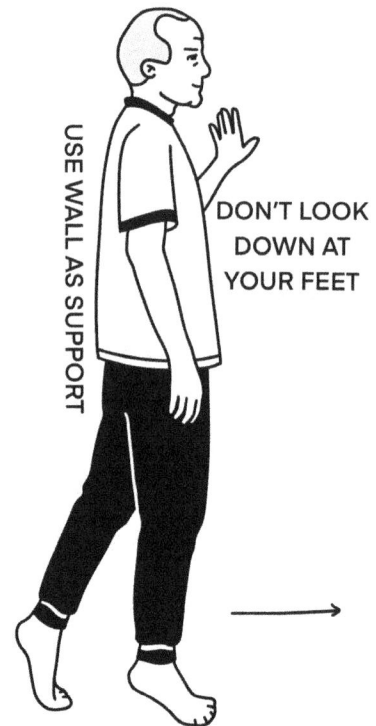

USE WALL AS SUPPORT

DON'T LOOK DOWN AT YOUR FEET

BREATHING

Maintain steady breathing throughout the whole exercise.

MODIFICATIONS

To **increase the challenge**, increase the speed or refrain from using the wall. To **decrease the challenge**, increase the amount of support from the wall.

TANDEM STANCE (WITH NECK ROTATION)

- Place a chair against a wall and stand facing the back of the chair while holding onto it with both hands.

- Place your feet in a tandem stance with the heel of one foot directly in front of the toes of the other foot.

- Let go of the chair and place your hands on your hips.

- Start turning your head to look to the left, come back through the center, and turn your head to the right.

- Try not to not use your hands if possible, but steady yourself on the back of the chair if needed.

- Keep your back straight and your shoulders relaxed.

- Maintain your balance with an equal amount of weight on both feet.

- Do not grip your toes.

- Repeat this exercise by alternating which foot is placed in front of the other.

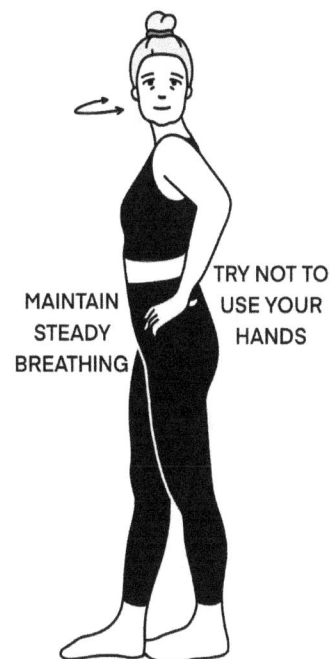

MAINTAIN STEADY BREATHING

TRY NOT TO USE YOUR HANDS

BREATHING

Maintain steady breathing throughout the whole exercise.

MODIFICATIONS

To **increase the challenge**, stand on a cushion. To **decrease the challenge**, widen your stance and keep your feet in a staggered position so that one isn't lined up directly behind the other, but a little bit to the side. You can also reduce the range in which you turn your neck.

FORWARD REACH (WITH A NARROW STANCE)

- Stand near a chair that is propped up against a wall or near a countertop.

- Place your feet side by side so they are touching each other.

- Keep your back straight and your shoulders relaxed.

- Place your hands straight out in front of you with your arms shoulder-width apart at shoulder height.

- Slowly shift your weight and reach forward as if reaching for something in front of you. Extend as far as you possibly can without falling forward.

- Return to a neutral position.

- Maintain your balance with an equal amount of weight on both feet.

- Do not grip your toes.

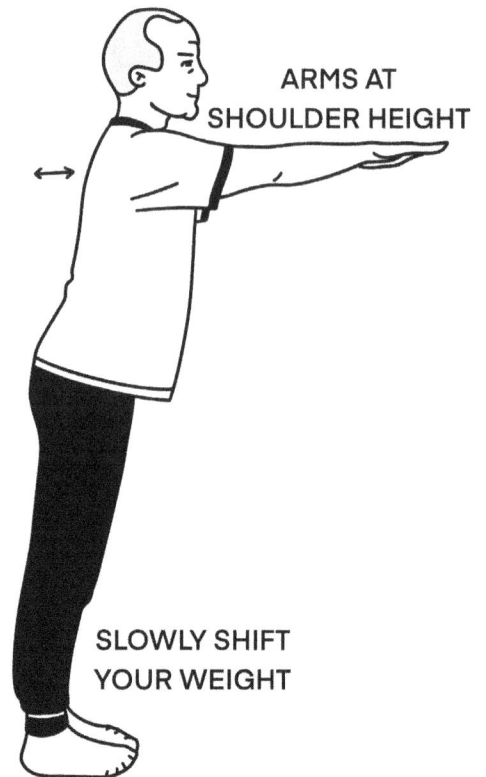

ARMS AT SHOULDER HEIGHT

SLOWLY SHIFT YOUR WEIGHT

BREATHING

Maintain steady breathing throughout the whole exercise.

MODIFICATIONS

To **increase the challenge**, stand on a cushion. To **decrease the challenge**, widen the space between your feet for more balance, or don't lean as far forward.

STANDING MARCH (WITHOUT SUPPORT)

- Stand near a chair that is propped up against a wall or near a countertop.

- Place your feet hip-distance apart.

- Keep your back straight and your shoulders relaxed.

- Engage your core.

- Lift one leg at a time to bring your hip and knee to a 90-degree angle.

- Maintain control as you alternate both legs for the recommended number of repetitions to mimic a marching movement.

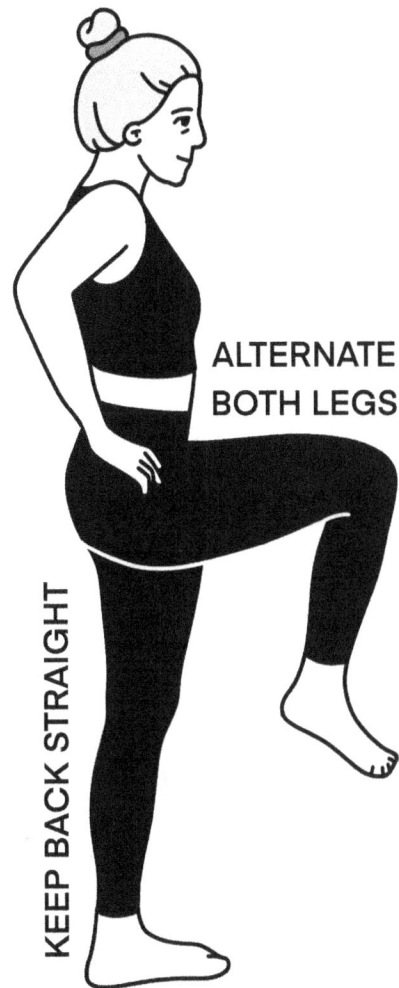

ALTERNATE BOTH LEGS

KEEP BACK STRAIGHT

BREATHING

Breathe in when you lift your knee towards your chest, and breathe out as you lower your knee.

MODIFICATIONS

To **increase the challenge**, add movement with the arms; when one knee lifts, the opposite arm moves up. To **decrease the challenge**, hold onto the back of a chair with one hand.

SIT-TO-STAND (WITH ONE LEG FORWARD)

- For this exercise, use a chair without armrests or refrain from using armrests, if your chair has them.

- Sit in an upright position toward the front of a chair and relax your shoulders.

- Place your feet hip-distance apart and flat on the floor.

- Now, slide one foot forward so that the heel of that foot is aligned with the toes of the other. Both toes should still be pointed forward.

- Extend your arms out in front of you at shoulder height.

- Lean your torso forward as you push into your feet and rise into a standing position.

- Maintain control as you reverse the motion and sit back down.

- Repeat ten times, then switch the foot position so the other one is more forward.

- The backward leg will be working harder during the exercise, but both feet should remain pressing into the floor.

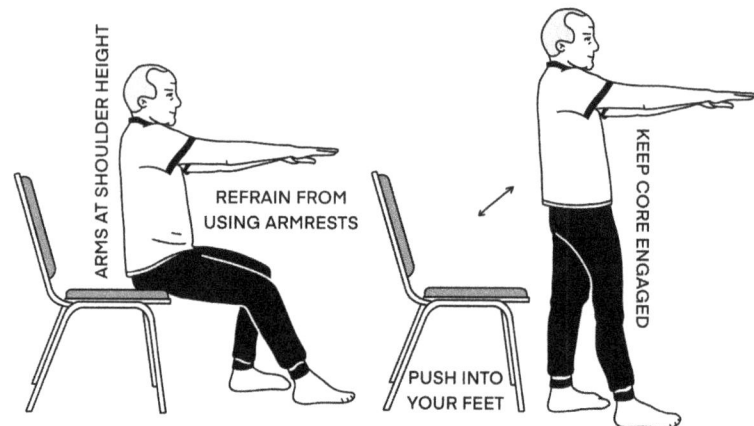

ARMS AT SHOULDER HEIGHT

REFRAIN FROM USING ARMRESTS

KEEP CORE ENGAGED

PUSH INTO YOUR FEET

BREATHING

Breathe in at the beginning of the movement to lengthen your spine, and breathe out as you move from sitting to standing. Breathe in as you sit back down.

MODIFICATIONS

To **increase the challenge**, cross your arms over your chest or use a lower chair. To **decrease the challenge**, place a cushion under your buttocks so you have less range of motion to cover, or hold onto the armrest with one hand.

HEEL WALKING

- Stand next to a wall with enough space to walk forward without any obstacles.

- Facing away from the wall, put one hand on the wall for support.

- Place your feet hip-distance apart.

- Keep your back straight and your shoulders relaxed.

- Shift your weight to the heels of both feet and lift the balls of the feet as high as possible. Be sure to keep your knees straight but not locked.

- Begin to walk forward keeping the front of the feet lifted.

- Look forward as you walk; do not look down at your feet.

- Release your feet back down to the floor after the recommended number of steps, turn around, and repeat by walking in the opposite direction.

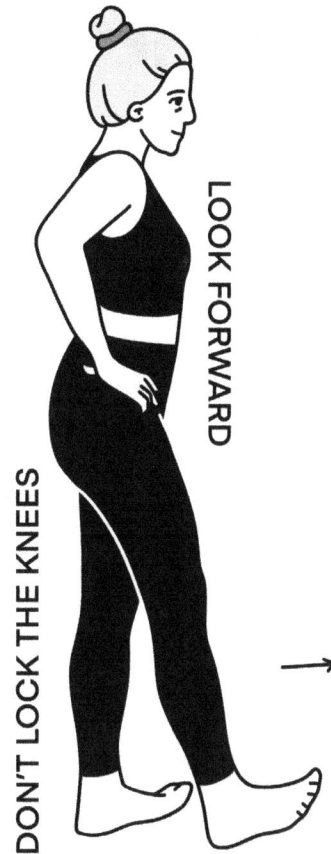

LOOK FORWARD

DON'T LOCK THE KNEES

BREATHING

Maintain steady breathing throughout the whole exercise.

MODIFICATIONS

To **increase the challenge**, increase the speed or refrain from using the wall. To **decrease the challenge**, increase the amount of support from the wall.

TANDEM HEEL-TO-TOE WALKING

- Stand next to a wall with enough space to walk forward without any obstacles.

- Facing away from the wall, put one hand on the wall for support.

- Keep your back straight and your shoulders relaxed.

- Place your feet in a tandem stance with the heel of one foot directly in front of the toes of the other foot.

- Begin to walk forward while alternating which foot is placed in front of the other.

- Do not grip your toes.

- Look forward as you walk; do not look down at your feet.

- After completing the recommended number of steps, turn around, and repeat by walking in the opposite direction.

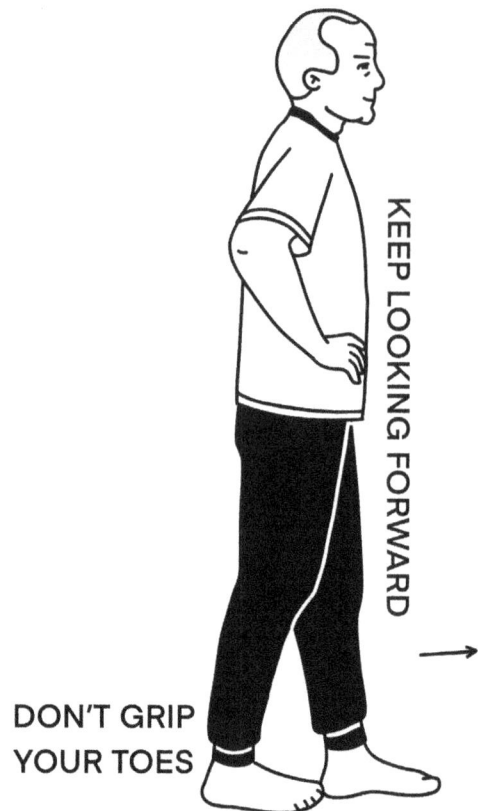

KEEP LOOKING FORWARD

DON'T GRIP YOUR TOES

BREATHING

Maintain steady breathing throughout the whole exercise.

MODIFICATIONS

To **increase the challenge**, increase the speed, refrain from using the wall, or rotate your head from left to right. To **decrease the challenge**, increase the amount of support from the wall or slightly widen your stance.

SQUAT (WITHOUT SUPPORT)

- Stand near a chair propped up against a wall or near a countertop.

- Place your feet hip-distance apart.

- Keep your back straight and your shoulders relaxed.

- Extend your arms out in front of you at shoulder height.

- Bend your knees and hips as if you were to sit back on a chair.

- Go as low as you can without feeling like you will fall backward.

- Keep equal weight on both feet.

- Slowly rise back up, extending the knees.

- Keep the entire foot flat on the floor for the duration of the exercise.

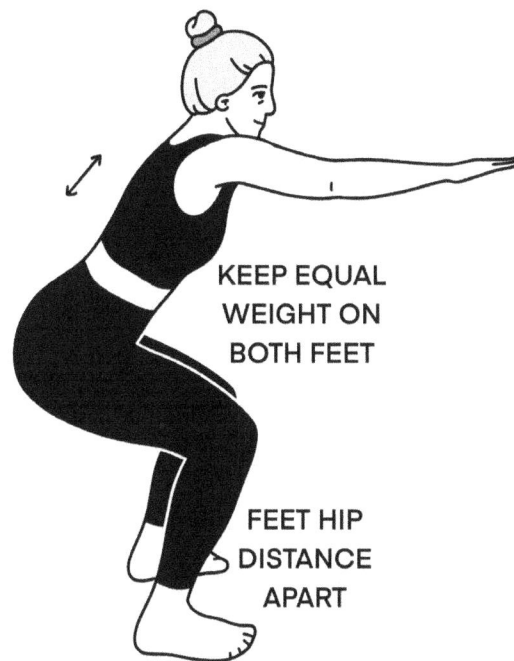

KEEP EQUAL WEIGHT ON BOTH FEET

FEET HIP DISTANCE APART

BREATHING

Breathe in when you bend your knees, and breathe out as you straighten your knees.

MODIFICATIONS

To **increase the challenge**, go deeper into the range of motion or cross your arms over your chest. To **decrease the challenge**, don't go as low when bending your knees or holding onto the back of the chair or countertop.

SINGLE-LEG STAND (WITH MOVEMENT OF FREE LEG)

- Place a chair against a wall and stand facing the back of the chair while holding onto it with both hands.

- Stand with your feet hip-distance apart.

- Keep your back straight and your shoulders relaxed.

- Bend one knee and lift your foot behind you, so that you are only standing on one leg.

- Let go of the chair and place your hands on your hips.

- Maintain your balance with the weight evenly distributed on the four corners of your foot.

- Begin moving your free leg back and forth to challenge your balance.

- Do not grip your toes.

- Repeat this exercise with your other foot.

- Try not to use your hands if possible, but you can catch your balance at any time by steadying yourself on the back of the chair if needed.

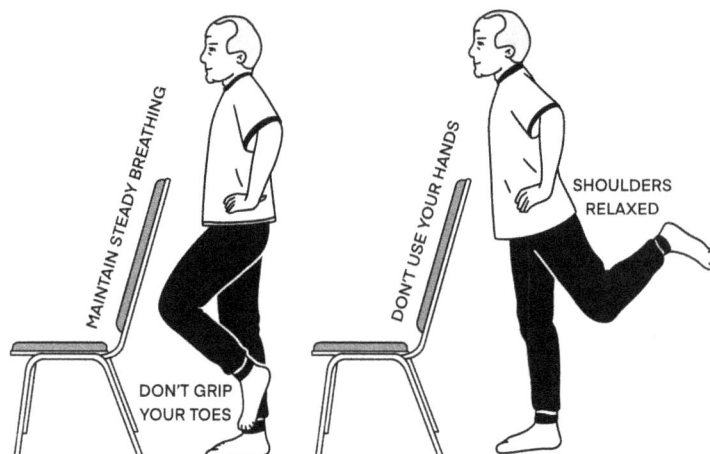

MAINTAIN STEADY BREATHING

DON'T GRIP YOUR TOES

DON'T USE YOUR HANDS

SHOULDERS RELAXED

BREATHING

Maintain steady breathing throughout the whole exercise.

MODIFICATIONS

To **increase the challenge**, stand on a cushion. To **decrease the challenge**, lightly hold onto the back of the chair for additional support.

SINGLE-LEG KNEE BEND (WITH LIGHT SUPPORT)

- Place a chair against a wall and stand with one hip facing the back of the chair while holding onto it with one hand.

- Your other hand can be on your hip furthest from the chair.

- Stand with your feet hip-distance apart.

- Keep your back straight and your shoulders relaxed.

- Bend one knee and lift your foot behind you, so that you are only standing on one leg.

- Bend your knee of the standing leg about 20-40 degrees.

- Control the motion and don't let the knee cave in toward the other leg.

- Push through your foot evenly to rise back up as you extend the knee.

- Do not grip your toes.

- Repeat this exercise with your other foot.

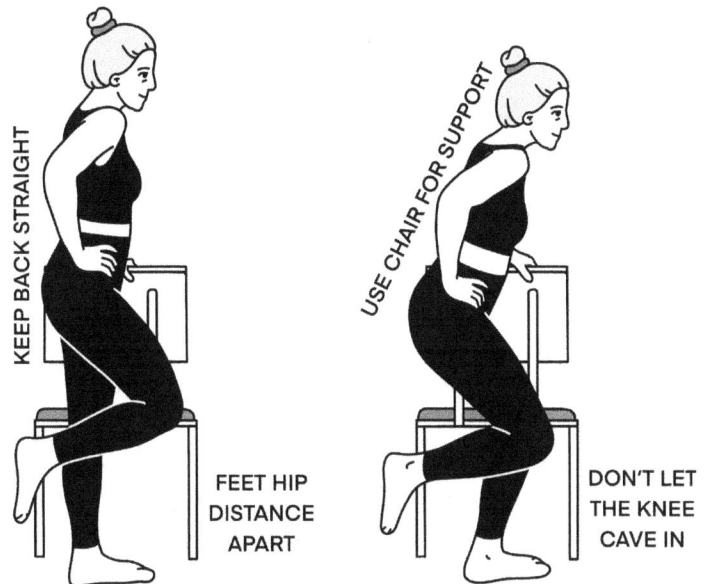

KEEP BACK STRAIGHT

FEET HIP DISTANCE APART

USE CHAIR FOR SUPPORT

DON'T LET THE KNEE CAVE IN

BREATHING

Maintain steady breathing throughout the whole exercise.

MODIFICATIONS

To **increase the challenge**, do not hold onto the chair, or only hold on it lightly. To **decrease the challenge**, decrease the range of motion when you bend your knee.

WALKING BACKWARD

- Stand next to a wall with enough space to walk backward without any obstacles.

- Facing away from the wall, put one hand on the wall for support.

- Keep your back straight and your shoulders relaxed.

- Begin to walk backward without trying to look over your shoulder.

- If possible, do not look down at your feet.

- After completing the recommended number of steps, turn around, and repeat by walking in the opposite direction.

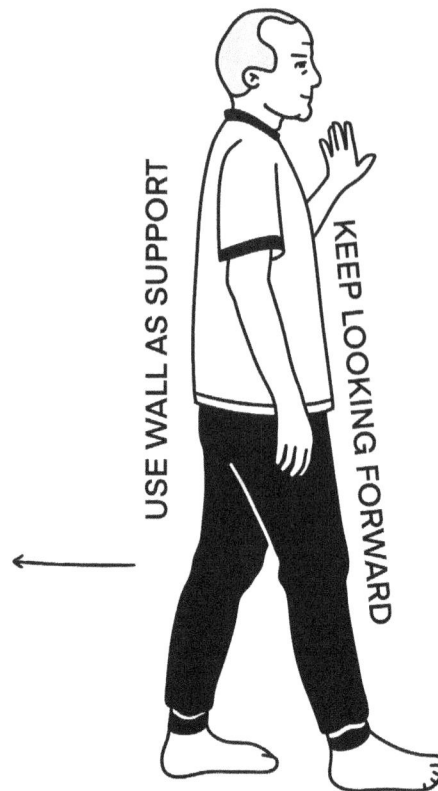

USE WALL AS SUPPORT

KEEP LOOKING FORWARD

BREATHING

Maintain steady breathing throughout the whole exercise.

MODIFICATIONS

To **increase the challenge**, increase the speed or refrain from using the wall. To **decrease the challenge**, increase the amount of support from the wall and slow down your speed.

28-DAY INTERMEDIATE-LEVEL BALANCE PLAN

Now that you have read through the **intermediate-level exercises for balance**, try to integrate these exercises into the following **28-day plan**. Use the following tables to keep yourself accountable and track your progress each week.

The plan is divided into **four weeks**; each week will get progressively more challenging. Please refer to the images and instructions to perform each exercise safely and correctly. Each week, you will perform **six exercises**. We recommend doing these **five or six times per week**. Include at least one rest day every week. If you follow the recommended number of repetitions, it should take 15 minutes or less to complete these balance exercises every day.

In addition to the exercises, we also recommend **walking for 30 minutes, at least five times per week**. You can divide your walking into separate sessions if you prefer doing so. For example, you could walk three times a day for 10 minutes, or two times a day for 15 minutes. Remember that every exercise session you complete is beneficial. Feel free to modify the recommended walking routine to best fit your individual needs.

You can walk without any assistance if you can do so safely, or use an assisted device such as a cane or a walker if needed. What is most important is that you stay safe and work within your limits.

INTERMEDIATE–LEVEL BALANCE EXERCISES

EXERCISE	REPETITIONS	DAY						
		MON	TUE	WED	THU	FRI	SAT	SUN
Unassisted sit–to–stand	10 reps (x2)							
Single–leg heel raises (with light support)	10 reps (x2)							
Side leg raises (with support)	15 reps (x2)							
Tandem stance (without support)	Hold for 10 (x3)							
Narrow stance (with neck rotation)	10 reps (x3)							
Single–leg stand (with support) Challenge: Perform without support	Hold for 10 (x3)							
Walking	30 minutes							

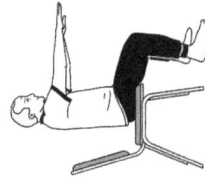

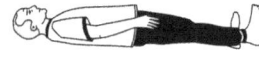

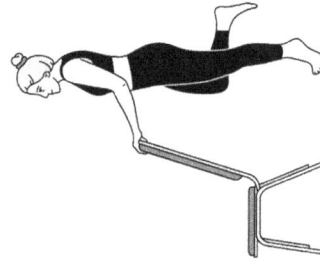

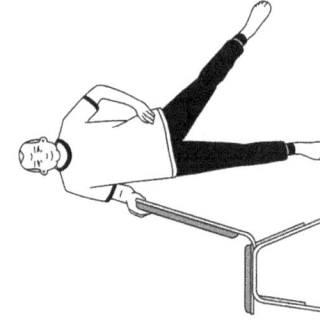

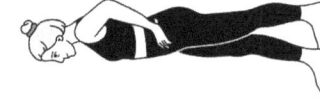

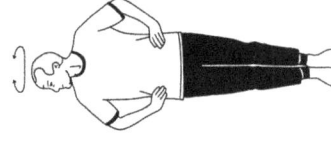

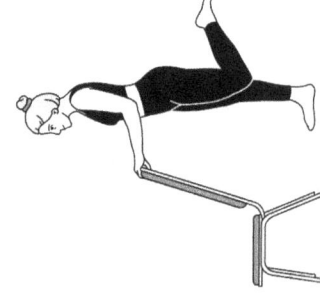

Unassisted sit–to–stand

Single–leg heel raises (with light support)

Side leg raises (with support)

Tandem stance (without support)

Narrow stance with neck rotation

Single–leg stand (with support)

INTERMEDIATE–LEVEL BALANCE EXERCISES

WEEK 2

EXERCISE	REPETITIONS	DAY						
		MON	TUE	WED	THU	FRI	SAT	SUN
Unassisted sit–to–stand	15 reps (x2)							
Toe walking	10 reps (x4)							
Side leg raises (with support) Challenge: Perform without support	10 reps (x2)							
Tandem stance (with neck rotation)	10 reps (x3)							
Forward reach (with narrow stance)	10 reps (x2)							
Standing march (without support)	20 reps (x2)							
Walking	30 minutes							

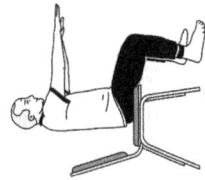

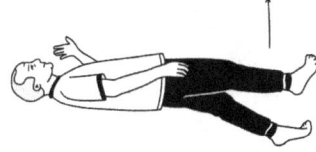

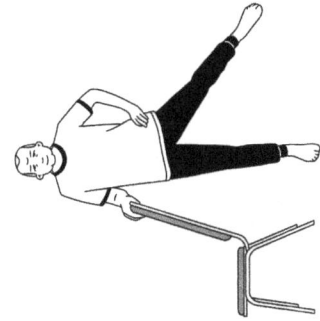

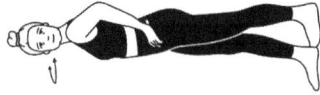

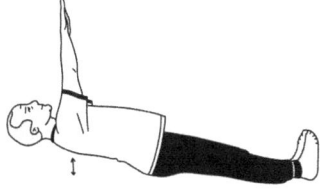

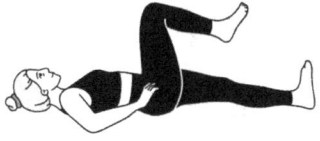

Unassisted sit–to–stand

Toe walking

Side leg raises (with support)

Tandem stance (with neck rotation)

Forward reach (with narrow stance)

Standing march (without support)

INTERMEDIATE-LEVEL BALANCE EXERCISES

EXERCISE	REPETITIONS	DAY						
		MON	TUE	WED	THU	FRI	SAT	SUN
Sit–to–stand (with one leg forward)	10 reps (x2)							
Heel walking	10 reps (x4)							
Tandem stance (without support) Challenge: Perform with a cushion	Hold for 10 (x3)							
Narrow stance (with neck rotation) Challenge: Perform with eyes closed	Hold for 10 (x3)							
Tandem heel–to–toe walking	10 reps (x4)							
Single–leg stand (without support) Challenge: Perform with a cushion.	Hold for 10 (x3)							
Walking	30 minutes							

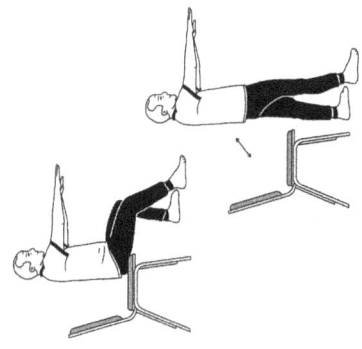

Sit–to–stand (with one leg forward)

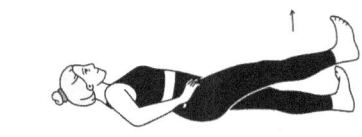

Heel walking

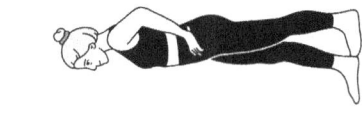

Tandem stance (without support)

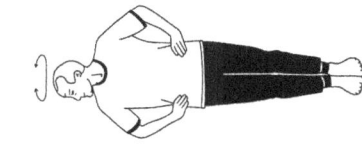

Narrow stance (with neck rotation)

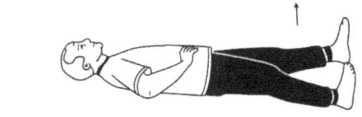

Tandem heel–to–toe walking

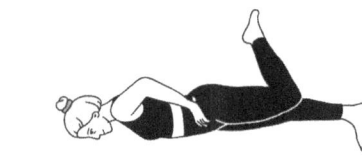

Single–leg stand (without support)

INTERMEDIATE-LEVEL BALANCE EXERCISES

EXERCISE	REPETITIONS	DAY						
		MON	TUE	WED	THU	FRI	SAT	SUN
Squat (without support)	10 reps (x2)							
Tandem Heel-To-Toe Walking Challenge: Perform rotating your head from left to right	10 reps (x4)							
Single-leg stand (with movement of free leg)	10 reps (x2)							
Single-leg knee bend (with light support)	10 reps (x2)							
Walking backward	10 reps (x4)							
Single-leg stand (without support) Challenge: Perform with eyes closed	Hold for 10 (x3)							
Walking	30 minutes							

Squat (without support)

Tandem Heel-To-Toe Walking

Single-leg stand (with movement of free leg)

single-leg knee bend (with light support)

Walking backward

single-leg stand (with eyes closed)

ADVANCED-LEVEL BALANCE EXERCISES

The advanced-level exercises have been selected to push the limits of your balance, coordination, and control.

These exercises include a greater range of movements that mimic movements commonly made throughout everyday activities.

You should be ready to practice the advanced-level exercises if you meet the following criteria:

- You have completed the intermediate-level program and are ready for a new challenge.

- You were at a **low risk of falling** when you completed your self-assessment for balance in Chapter 3.

If you are a complete beginner, you should begin with either the beginner or intermediate exercises before proceeding to the advanced-level exercises. This level is designed to push the limits of your balance skills, if practiced regularly. Each exercise includes modifications so that you may adapt the exercise to fit your comfort level.

Some of these exercises will suggest you use a prop like a cushion, or close your eyes to challenge your balance. Please remember that it's always optional and isn't a requirement if you don't feel comfortable or safe doing so.

Following the list of advanced exercises, you will find a 28-day plan that gradually integrates each of these exercises. This will help you reach the SMART balance goal that you have set in Chapter 6.

SQUAT (WITHOUT SUPPORT)

- Stand near a chair propped up against a wall or near a countertop, in case you need support.

- Place your feet hip-distance apart.

- Keep your back straight and your shoulders relaxed.

- Extend your arms out in front of you at shoulder height.

- Bend your knees and hips as if you were to sit back on a chair.

- Go as low as you can without feeling like you will fall backward.

- Keep equal weight on both feet.

- Slowly rise back up, extending the knees.

- Keep the entire foot flat on the floor for the duration of the exercise.

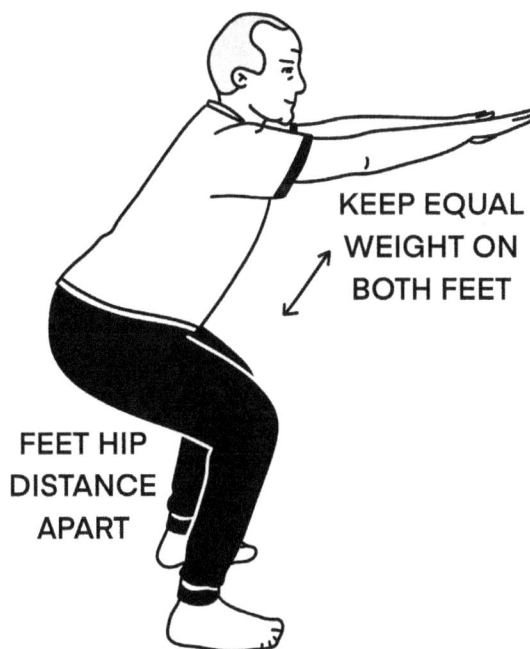

KEEP EQUAL WEIGHT ON BOTH FEET

FEET HIP DISTANCE APART

BREATHING

Breathe in when you bend your knees, and breathe out as you straighten you knees.

MODIFICATIONS

To **increase the challenge**, go deeper into the range of motion, cross your arms over your chest or stand on a cushion. To **decrease the challenge**, don't go as low when bending your knees or hold onto the back of the chair for support.

TANDEM WALKING (WITH NECK ROTATION)

- Stand next to a wall with enough space to walk forward without any obstacles.

- Facing away from the wall, put one hand on the wall for support.

- Keep your back straight and your shoulders relaxed.

- Place your feet in a tandem stance with the heel of one foot directly in front of the toes of the other foot.

- Begin to walk forward while alternating which foot is placed in front of the other.

- At the same time, slowly rotate your head to look from left to right.

- Do not grip your toes.

- After completing ten steps, turn around, and repeat going back the other way.

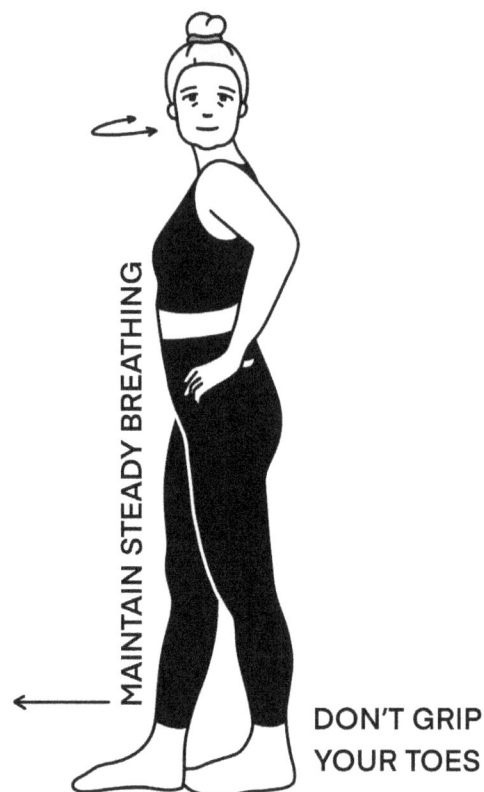

MAINTAIN STEADY BREATHING

DON'T GRIP YOUR TOES

BREATHING

Maintain steady breathing throughout the whole exercise.

MODIFICATIONS

To **increase the challenge**, increase the speed, and refrain from using the wall for support. To **decrease the challenge**, increase the amount of support from the wall or slightly widen the stance.

SINGLE-LEG STAND (WITH ARM MOVEMENT)

- Place a chair against a wall and stand facing the back of the chair while holding onto it with both hands.

- Stand with your feet hip-distance apart.

- Keep your back straight and your shoulders relaxed.

- Bend one knee and lift your foot behind you, so that you are only standing on one leg.

- Let go of the chair and place your hands by your side.

- Maintain your balance with the weight evenly distributed on the four corners of your foot.

- Begin moving your arms up and down alternating the left and the right side.

- Do not grip your toes.

- Repeat this exercise with your other foot.

- If needed, use the chair to help you catch your balance.

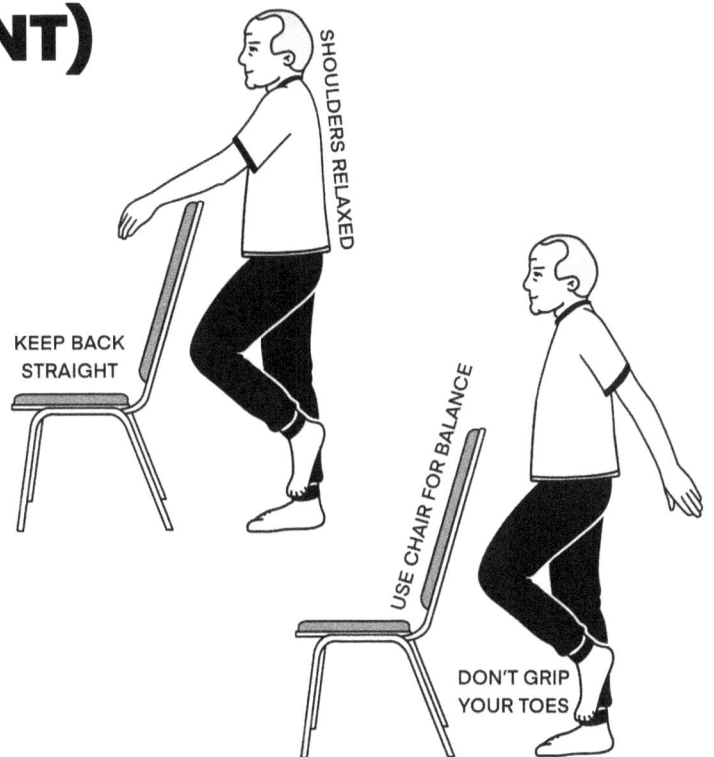

BREATHING

Maintain steady breathing throughout the whole exercise.

MODIFICATIONS

To **increase the challenge**, stand on a cushion. To **decrease the challenge**, lightly touch the toes of your free leg on the floor for additional support.

MINI LUNGE (STAGGERED STANCE WITH KNEE BEND)

- Place a chair against a wall and stand so that one of your hips is near the back of the chair.

- Place your feet hip-distance apart.

- Take a step forward with your right foot.

- Keep your back straight and your shoulders relaxed.

- Bend both knees about 20-40 degrees.

- Don't let the front knee cave in.

- The heel of the back foot lifts from the floor while the front foot stays anchored to the floor.

- Slowly extend both knees to stand tall once again.

- Alternate which foot is forward, and repeat movement.

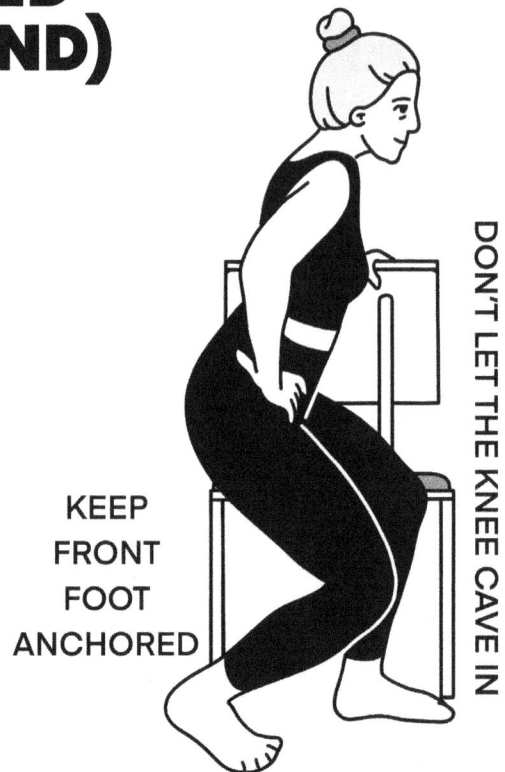

KEEP FRONT FOOT ANCHORED

DON'T LET THE KNEE CAVE IN

BREATHING

Breathe in as you bend both knees and breathe out as you extend your knees.

MODIFICATIONS

To **increase the challenge**, increase the bend in the knees or stand on a cushion. To **decrease the challenge**, hold onto the chair with one hand.

WALKING SIDE-TO-SIDE

- Stand facing a wall with enough space to walk side-to-side without any obstacles.

- Bring your hands out in front of you for safety in case you lose your balance.

- Start with your feet together.

- Keep your back straight and your shoulders relaxed.

- Decide which way you want to go first and take a step in that direction.

- Immediately follow the movement with your other foot so both feet can join.

- If possible, do not look down at your feet.

- Keep stepping from side-to-side.

- After completing the recommended number of steps, pause, and repeat by moving in the opposite direction.

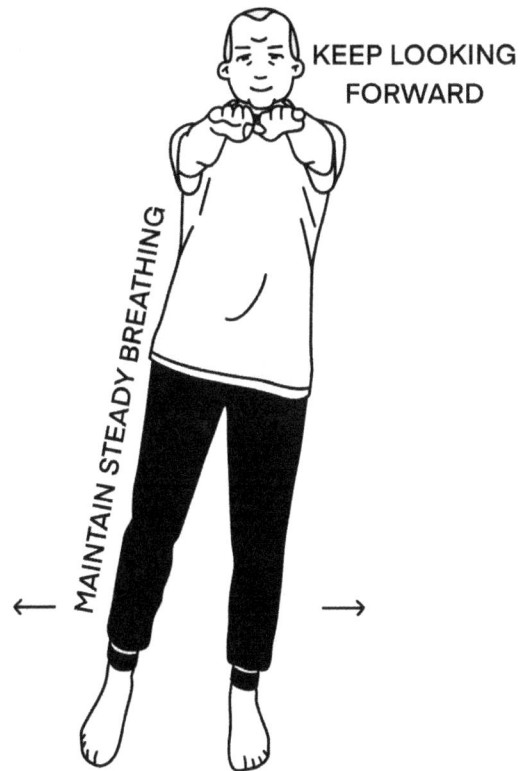

KEEP LOOKING FORWARD

MAINTAIN STEADY BREATHING

BREATHING

Maintain steady breathing throughout the whole exercise.

MODIFICATIONS

To **increase the challenge**, increase the speed of your walking. To **decrease the challenge**, place one hand against the wall for support, or decrease your speed.

SINGLE-LEG KNEE BEND (WITH LIGHT SUPPORT)

- Place a chair against a wall and stand with one hip facing the back of the chair while holding onto it with one hand.

- Your other hand can be on your hip.

- Stand with your feet hip-distance apart.

- Keep your back straight and your shoulders relaxed.

- Bend one knee and lift your foot behind you, so that you are only standing on one leg.

- Bend your knee of the standing leg about 20-40 degrees.

- Control the motion and don't let the knee lean toward the other leg.

- Push through your foot evenly to rise back up as you extend the knee.

- Do not grip your toes.

- Repeat this exercise with your other foot.

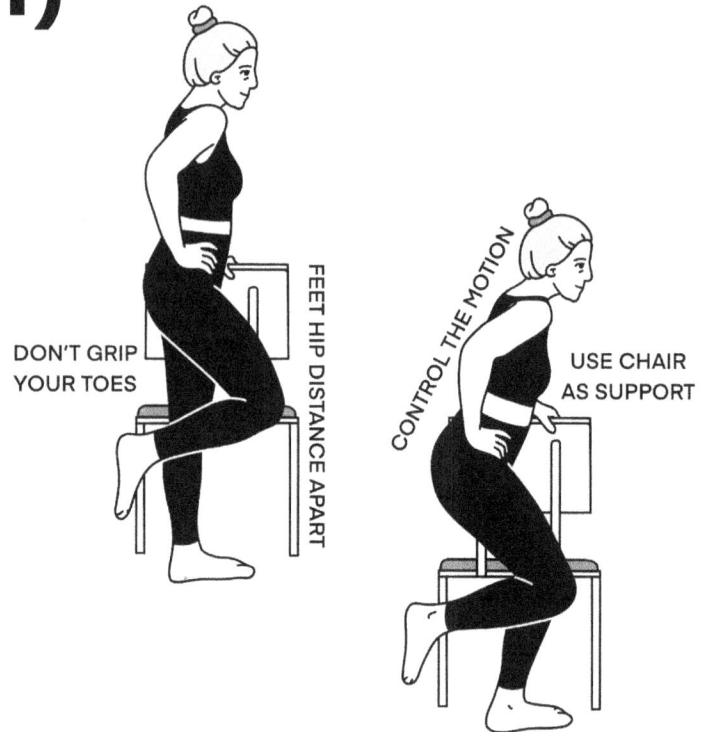

DON'T GRIP YOUR TOES

FEET HIP DISTANCE APART

CONTROL THE MOTION

USE CHAIR AS SUPPORT

BREATHING

Maintain steady breathing throughout the whole exercise.

MODIFICATIONS

To **increase the challenge**, do not use support, stand on a cushion, or close your eyes. To **decrease the challenge**, decrease the range of motion when you bend your knee.

SINGLE-LEG STAND (WITH EYE MOVEMENT)

- Stand next to a chair propped against a wall or a countertop.

- Stand with your feet hip-distance apart.

- Keep your back straight and your shoulders relaxed.

- Bend one knee and lift your foot behind you, so that you are only standing on one leg.

- Place one hand on your hip and lift your other arm so your index finger is at eye level.

- Maintain your balance with the weight evenly distributed on the four corners of your foot.

- Slowly move your index finger from left to right about 3 inches maximum on each side.

- Follow your finger with your eyes, but don't move your head or your trunk.

- Do not grip your toes.

- Repeat this exercise with your other foot.

- The chair is there to help you catch your balance at any time if needed.

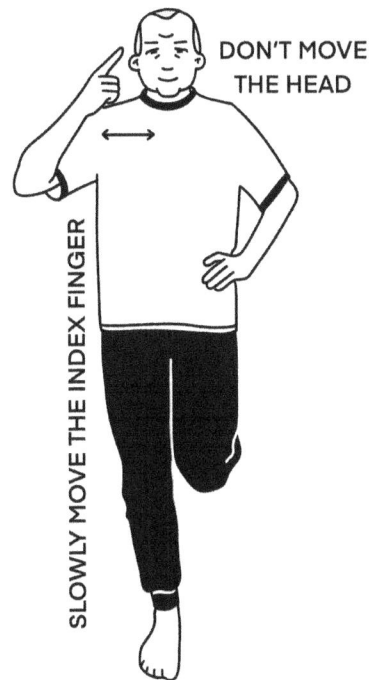

DON'T MOVE THE HEAD

SLOWLY MOVE THE INDEX FINGER

BREATHING

Maintain steady breathing throughout the whole exercise.

MODIFICATIONS

To **increase the challenge**, stand on a cushion. To **decrease the challenge**, lightly touch the toes of your free leg on the floor or hold onto the chair with one hand for additional support.

TANDEM TOE-TO-HEEL WALKING (BACKWARD)

- Stand next to a wall with enough space to walk backward without any obstacles.

- Facing away from the wall, put one hand on the wall for support.

- Keep your back straight and your shoulders relaxed.

- Place your feet in a tandem stance with the heel of one foot directly in front of the toes of the other foot.

- Begin to walk backward while alternating which foot is placed behind the other.

- Do not grip your toes.

- Look forward as you walk; do not look down at your feet.

- After completing the recommended number of steps, turn around, walk in the opposite direction.

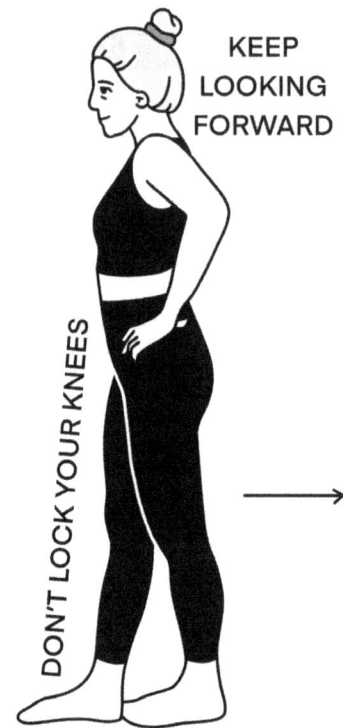

KEEP LOOKING FORWARD

DON'T LOCK YOUR KNEES

BREATHING

Maintain steady breathing throughout the whole exercise.

MODIFICATIONS

To **increase the challenge**, increase the speed, refrain from using the wall, or add some head turns from left to right. To **decrease the challenge**, increase the amount of support from the wall or slightly widen the stance.

360-DEGREE TURN

- Stand near a chair propped up against a wall or near a countertop, in case you need support.

- Place your feet hip-distance apart.

- Keep your back straight and your shoulders relaxed.

- Choose which direction you want to turn in.

- Begin taking small steps to turn in one direction until you face back the same way again.

- Take a small pause and make sure to reposition your feet at hip-distance apart.

- Repeat the same movement in the other direction.

- Keep your head in line with your spine and avoid looking at your feet.

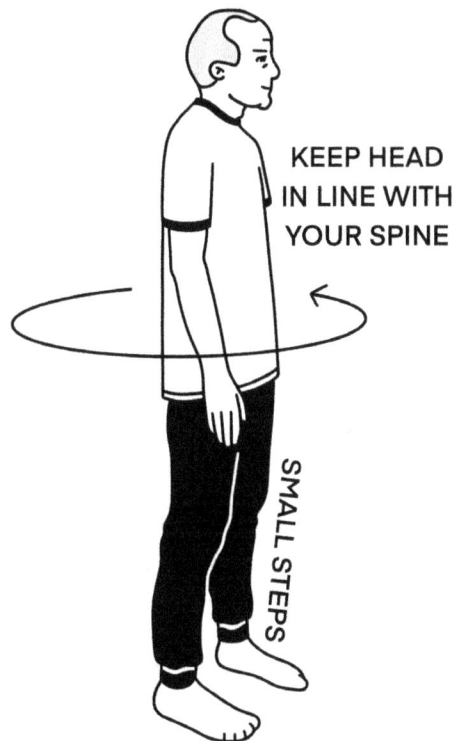

KEEP HEAD IN LINE WITH YOUR SPINE

SMALL STEPS

BREATHING

Maintain steady breathing throughout the whole exercise.

MODIFICATIONS

To **increase the challenge**, increase the speed at which you turn. To **decrease the challenge**, widen your stance even more and slow down the speed at which you turn.

SQUAT HOLD (WITHOUT SUPPORT)

- Stand near a chair propped up against a wall or near a countertop.

- Place your feet hip-distance apart.

- Keep your back straight and your shoulders relaxed.

- Extend your arms out in front of you at shoulder height.

- Bend your knees and hips as if you were to sit back on a chair.

- Go as low as you can while still maintaining control, then hold the position at the bottom of the squat.

- Keep equal weight on both feet.

- Hold for the recommended amount of time before rising back up.

- Keep the entire foot flat on the floor for the duration of the exercise.

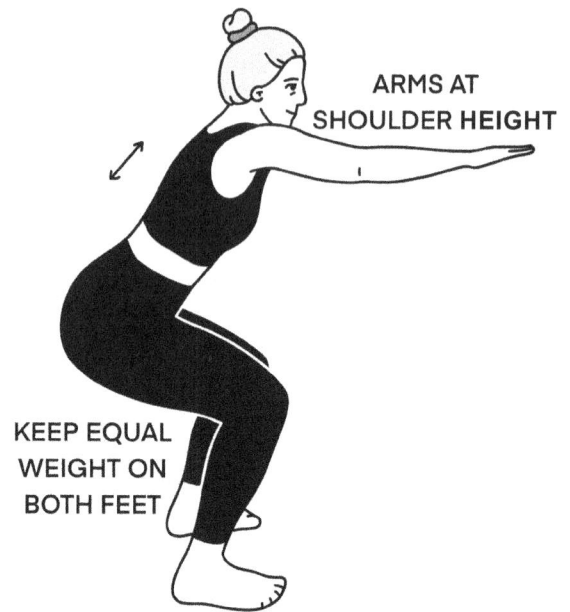

ARMS AT SHOULDER HEIGHT

KEEP EQUAL WEIGHT ON BOTH FEET

BREATHING

Maintain steady breathing throughout the whole exercise.

MODIFICATIONS

To **increase the challenge**, go deeper into the range of motion or stand on a cushion. To **decrease the challenge**, modify your knee bend, or lightly hold onto the back of the chair or countertop.

SINGLE-LEG STAND (WITH EYES CLOSED)

- Place a chair against a wall and stand facing the back of the chair while holding onto it with both hands.

- Stand with your feet hip-distance apart.

- Keep your back straight and your shoulders relaxed.

- Bend one knee and lift your foot behind you, so that you are only standing on one leg.

- Let go of the chair and place your hands on your hips.

- Maintain your balance with the weight evenly distributed on the four corners of your foot.

- Close your eyes.

- Do not grip your toes.

- Repeat this exercise with your other foot.

- Try not using your hands, but you can catch your balance at any time with the back of the chair if needed.

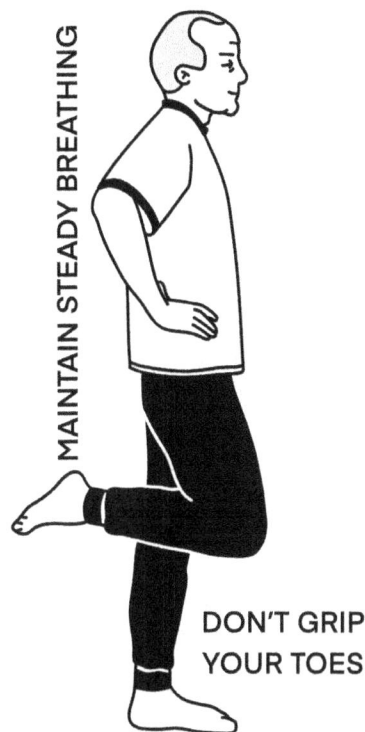

MAINTAIN STEADY BREATHING

DON'T GRIP YOUR TOES

BREATHING

Maintain steady breathing throughout the whole exercise.

MODIFICATIONS

To **increase the challenge**, stand on a cushion. To **decrease the challenge**, lightly rest the toes of your raised foot on the floor or rest your hands on the back of the chair to steady yourself.

TANDEM HEEL-TO-TOE WALKING (WITH A MENTAL TASK)

- Stand next to a wall with enough space to walk forward without any obstacles.

- Facing away from the wall, put one hand on the wall for support.

- Keep your back straight and your shoulders relaxed.

- Place your feet in a tandem stance with the heel of one foot directly in front of the toes of the other foot.

- Begin to walk forward while alternating which foot is placed in front of the other.

- At the same time, count backward from a hundred.

- Do not grip your toes.

- Look forward as you walk; do not look down at your feet.

- After completing ten steps, repeat in the opposite direction.

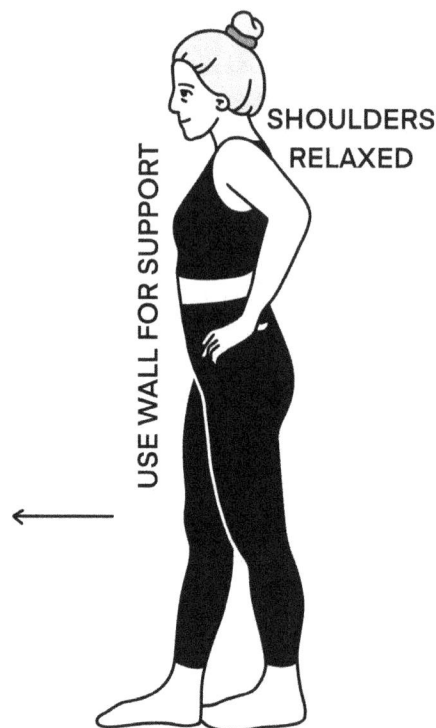

USE WALL FOR SUPPORT

SHOULDERS RELAXED

BREATHING

Maintain steady breathing throughout the whole exercise.

MODIFICATIONS

To **increase the challenge**, increase the speed, refrain from using the wall. To **decrease the challenge**, increase the amount of support from the wall or slightly widen your stance.

SQUAT-TO-HEEL RAISES (WITHOUT SUPPORT)

- Stand near a chair propped up against a wall or near a countertop, in case you need support.

- Place your feet hip-distance apart.

- Keep your back straight and your shoulders relaxed.

- Extend your arms out in front of you at shoulder height.

- Bend your knees and hips as if you were to sit back on a chair.

- Go as low as you can without feeling like you will fall backward.

- Keep equal weight on both feet.

- Slowly rise back up, extending the knees.

- Lift your heels from the floor to stand on the balls of your feet.

- Alternate slowly between these two movements for the recommended number of repetitions.

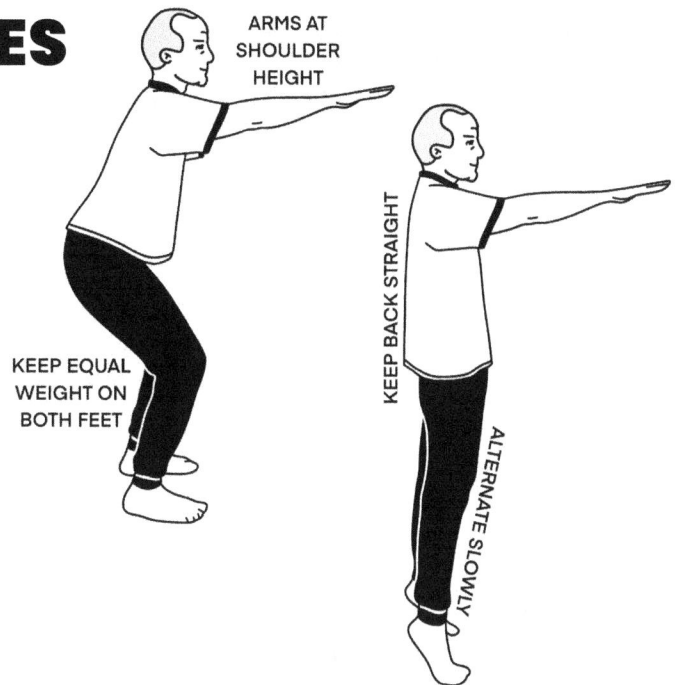

ARMS AT SHOULDER HEIGHT

KEEP EQUAL WEIGHT ON BOTH FEET

KEEP BACK STRAIGHT

ALTERNATE SLOWLY

BREATHING

Breathe in when you bend your knees, and breathe out as you straighten your knees. Breathe in when you lift your heels, and breathe out when you bring your heels back down.

MODIFICATIONS

To **increase the challenge**, go deeper into your squat or cross your arms over your chest. To **decrease the challenge**, don't go as low into your squat and heel raise, or lightly hold onto the back of the chair or countertop.

SINGLE-LEG STAND (WITH TORSO ROTATION)

- Stand near a chair propped up against a wall or near a countertop and hold onto it.

- Stand with your feet hip-distance apart.

- Keep your back straight and your shoulders relaxed.

- Bend one knee and lift your foot behind you, so that you are only standing on one leg.

- Let go of the chair and cross your arms over your chest.

- Maintain your balance with the weight evenly distributed on the four corners of your foot.

- Turn your torso to one side, come back to the center, and then turn to the other side.

- Turn at about 45 degrees on each side.

- Do not grip your toes.

- Repeat this exercise with your other foot.

- If possible, do not use your hands, but catch your balance with the back of the chair if needed.

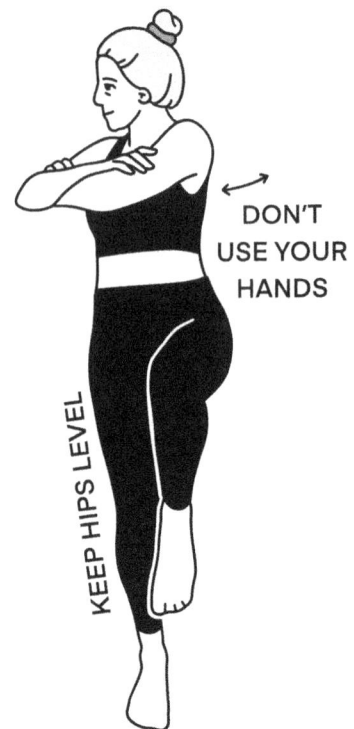

DON'T USE YOUR HANDS

KEEP HIPS LEVEL

BREATHING

Maintain steady breathing throughout the whole exercise.

MODIFICATIONS

To **increase the challenge**, stand on a cushion. To **decrease the challenge**, lightly rest the toes of your raised foot on the floor or reduce the range of motion during each torso rotation.

STANDING MARCH (WITH PAUSES)

- Stand near a chair that is propped up against a wall or near a countertop.

- Place your feet hip-distance apart.

- Keep your back straight and your shoulders relaxed.

- Engage your core.

- Lift one leg at a time to bring your hip and knee to a 90-degree angle.

- Pause at the top of the movement for 2 seconds.

- Lower the leg back toward the floor.

- Maintain control as you alternate both legs for the recommended number of repetitions to mimic a marching movement.

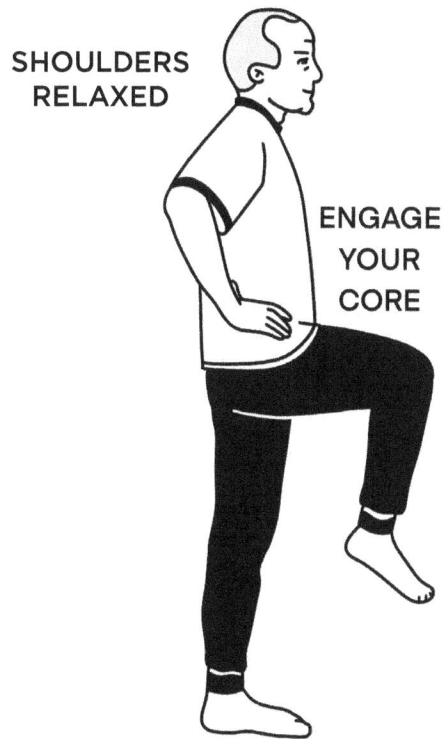

SHOULDERS RELAXED

ENGAGE YOUR CORE

BREATHING

Breathe in when you lift your knee towards your chest, and breathe out as you lower your knee.

MODIFICATIONS

To **increase the challenge**, add movement of the arms; when the left knee lifts, the right arm moves up. To **decrease the challenge**, hold onto the back of a chair or countertop with one hand.

WALKING BACKWARD (WITH NECK ROTATION)

- Stand next to a wall with enough space to walk backward without any obstacles.

- Facing away from the wall, put one hand on the wall for support.

- Keep your back straight and your shoulders relaxed.

- Begin to walk backward.

- At the same time, slowly rotate your head from left to right.

- If possible, do not look down at your feet.

- After completing the recommended number of steps, repeat in the opposite direction.

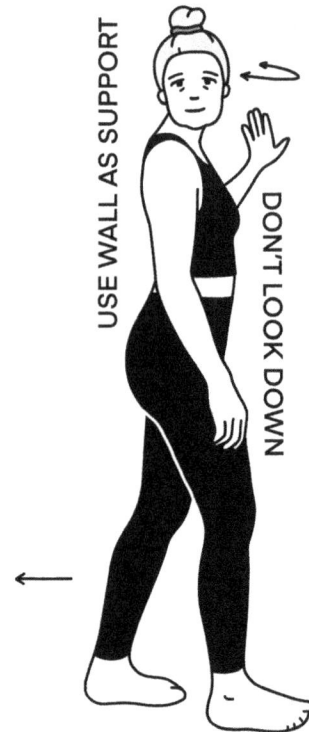

USE WALL AS SUPPORT

DON'T LOOK DOWN

BREATHING

Maintain steady breathing throughout the whole exercise.

MODIFICATIONS

To **increase the challenge**, increase the speed or refrain from using the wall. To **decrease the challenge**, use the wall for support and slow down your speed.

ALTERNATING TOE TAPS (ON A STEP)

- Stand near a countertop in case you need support.

- Place a small (eight or nine inch high) step against the wall in front of the countertop.

- Place your feet hip-distance apart.

- Keep your back straight and your shoulders relaxed.

- Engage your core.

- Lift one leg at a time to tap the front of your foot onto the step.

- Maintain control as you alternate both feet for the recommended number of repetitions.

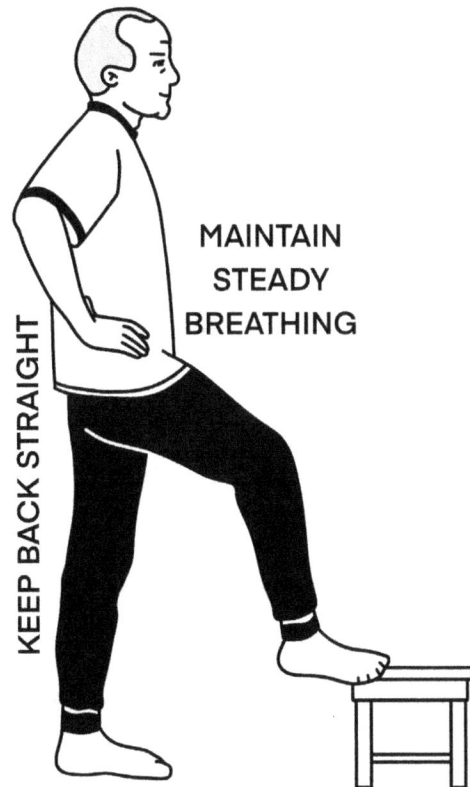

KEEP BACK STRAIGHT

MAINTAIN STEADY BREATHING

BREATHING

Maintain steady breathing throughout the whole exercise.

MODIFICATIONS

To **increase the challenge**, increase your speed as you tap your feet on the step. To **decrease the challenge**, hold onto a countertop for support.

28-DAY ADVANCED-LEVEL BALANCE PLAN

Now that you have read through the **advanced-level exercises for balance**, try to integrate these exercises into the following **28-day plan**. Use the following tables to keep yourself accountable and track your progress each week.

The plan is divided into **four weeks**; each week will get progressively more challenging. Please refer to the images and instructions to safely and correctly perform each exercise. Each week, you will perform **six exercises**.

We recommend doing these **five or six times per week**. Include at least one rest day every week. If you follow the recommended number of repetitions, it should take 15 minutes or less to complete these balance exercises every day.

In addition to the exercises, we also recommend **walking for 30 minutes, at least 5 times per week**. Remember that every exercise session you complete is beneficial. You can divide your walking into separate sessions if you prefer doing so. For example, you could walk three times a day for 10 minutes, or two times a day for 15 minutes.

Feel free to modify the recommended walking routine to best fit your individual needs. You can walk without any assistance if you can do so safely, or use an assisted device such as a cane or a walker if needed. What is most important is that you stay safe and work within your limits.

ADVANCED-LEVEL BALANCE EXERCISES

EXERCISE	REPETITIONS	DAY						
		MON	TUE	WED	THU	FRI	SAT	SUN
Squat (without support)	10 reps (x2)							
Tandem walking (with neck rotation)	10 reps (x4)							
Single-leg stand (with arm movement)	10 reps (x2)							
Mini lunge (staggered stance with knee bend)	10 reps (x2)							
Walking side-to-side	10 reps (x4)							
Single-leg knee bend (with light support)	Hold for 10 (x3)							
Walking	30 minutes							

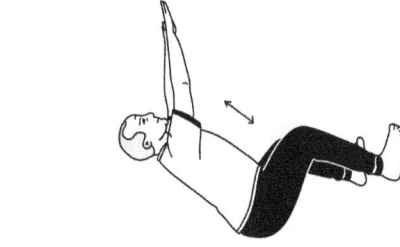

Squat (without support)

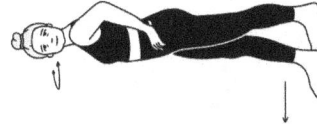

Tandem walking (with neck rotation)

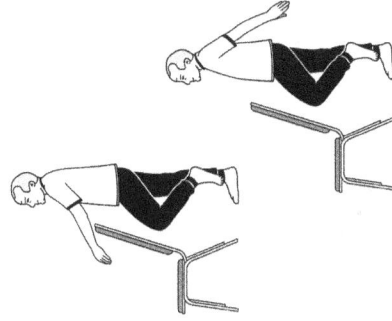

Single-leg stand (with arm movement)

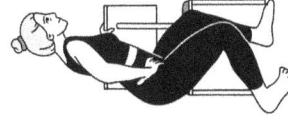

Mini lunge (staggered stance with knee bend)

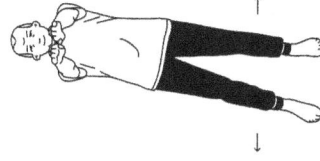

Walking side-to-side

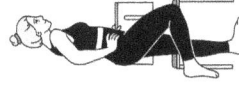

Single-leg knee bend (with light support)

ADVANCED-LEVEL BALANCE EXERCISES

EXERCISE	REPETITIONS	DAY						
		MON	TUE	WED	THU	FRI	SAT	SUN
Squat (without support) Challenge: Perform with a cushion	10 reps (x2)							
Single-leg stand (with eye movement)	10 reps (x2)							
Mini lunge (staggered stance with knee bend)	15 reps (x2)							
Tandem toe-to-heel walking (backward)	10 reps (x4)							
360-degree turn	10 reps (each direction)							
Single-leg knee bend (with light support) Challenge: Do not use support	10 reps (x2)							
Walking	30 minutes							

Squat (without support)

Single-leg stand (with eye movement)

Mini lunge (staggered stance with knee bend)

Tandem toe-to-heel walking (backward)

360-degree turn

Single-leg knee bend (with light support)

ADVANCED–LEVEL BALANCE EXERCISES

WEEK 3

EXERCISE	REPETITIONS	DAY						
		MON	TUE	WED	THU	FRI	SAT	SUN
Squat hold (without support) Challenge: Do not use support	Hold for 10 (x5)							
Single–leg stand (with eyes closed)	10 reps (x2)							
Mini lunge (staggered stance with knee bend) Challenge: Perform with a cushion	10 reps (x2)							
Tandem heel–to–toe walking (with a mental task)	10 reps (x4)							
Squat to heel raises (without support)	10 reps (x2)							
Single–leg knee bend (with light support) Challenge: Do not use support and use a cushion	10 reps (x2)							
Walking	30 minutes							

squat hold (without support)

single–leg stand (with eyes closed)

Mini lunge (staggered stance with knee bend)

Tandem heel–to–toe walking (with a mental task)

Squat to heel raises (without support)

Single–leg knee bend (with light support)

ADVANCED–LEVEL BALANCE EXERCISES

EXERCISE	REPETITIONS	DAY						
		MON	TUE	WED	THU	FRI	SAT	SUN
Squat (without support) Challenge: Do not use support and use a cushion	Hold for 10 (x5)							
Single-leg stand (with torso rotation)	10 reps (x2)							
Single-leg knee bend (with light support) Challenge: Do not use support and use a cushion.	10 reps (x2)							
Standing march (with pauses)	20 alternating marches (x2)							
Walking backward (with neck rotation)	10 reps (x4)							
Alternating toe taps (on a step)	20 alternating marches (x2)							
Walking	30 minutes							

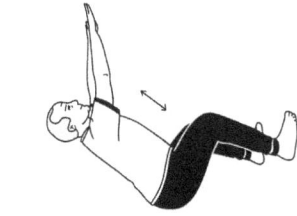

Squat (without support)

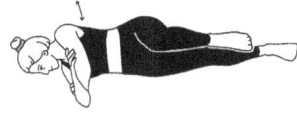

Single-leg stand (with torso rotation)

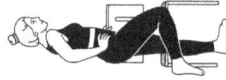

Single-leg knee bend (with light support)

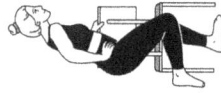

Standing march (with pause)

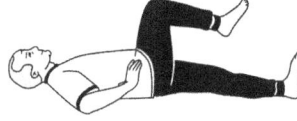

Walking backward (with neck rotation)

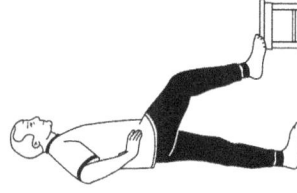

Alternating toe taps (on a step)

CHAPTER 8

MAINTAINING BALANCE BEYOND THE BASICS

To ensure that you keep improving your balance, it's important that you stay consistent with your balance exercises. Even after you finish the 28-day plan, it's important to continue to practice the balance exercises you have learned.

You might choose to complete another 28-day plan at a more challenging level. Or, you could repeat week 4 of your 28-day plan until you feel more confident in your abilities. At some point, your goal might be to simply maintain your balancing abilities instead of improving. In this case, you might choose to repeat the advanced exercises for week 4, or vary the exercises in a way that keeps you feeling challenged. What is most important is that you stay consistent and keep putting in the effort to do your balance exercises to improve or maintain your progress.

HOW TO TRACK YOUR PROGRESS

As you learned earlier, it's never too late to learn new skills and you can still boost your performance as you get older. Your balance is a skill that can still be improved and the only way to improve it is to keep working on it. To stay motivated in doing so and to see if your balance routine is effective, it's important to track your progress.

Here are a few tips that can help you track your progress over time:

1. **Do the balance self-assessment every 4 to 6 weeks.**

   You can always come back to the self-assessments to see how you are progressing. Make sure you keep a log of your test results with the date so you can compare them over time. You won't necessarily notice massive improvements every time you do the self-assessment and that is all right. As long as you keep challenging yourself enough with the exercises, you are on the right path.

It's also possible that at some point you no longer have the desire or need to improve if you have reached your goal. You can simply keep doing your balance exercises to maintain your abilities. In this case, your test results should remain stable. However, if you are doing the balance exercises and notice a decline in your results time after time, it can be a good idea to consult with a healthcare professional for more structured guidance.

2. Keep a journal or log of your balance exercise routine.

Another great way to track your progress is to keep a log of your workouts. Write down the name of the exercises, the date, the number of sets and reps, as well as how challenging the session was. Keep it simple by writing down if the exercise session was easy, medium, or difficult.

If you find yourself always writing that it's easy, this could be a good indicator that you need to challenge yourself further. On the other hand, if you notice that you are feeling drained from your balance routines and that it's often feeling difficult, it might be wise to decrease the intensity.

3. Get visual feedback.

Another tip to track your progression is to ask a family member or a friend to record you. For example, if part of your goal is to improve your ability to walk, you can ask someone to take a video of you walking. After working on your balance for 4-6 weeks, ask them to take another video to see if you notice any improvements.

After doing the balance exercises you might feel like you are more confident or steady on your feet. Having visual proof from a video can help validate how you feel and give you objective proof that you are improving.

The main takeaway is to not give up on your balance exercise routine. Maintain your good habits by investing 15 minutes out of every day to work on balance and encourage yourself to keep going. We'll discuss ways to adapt and modify the exercises to ensure that they remain safe and efficient throughout your practice.

CHAPTER 9

ADAPTATIONS AND MODIFICATIONS

Earlier, we mentioned the importance of self-assessment for balance which will give you an idea about your balancing abilities and your risk of falling. By undergoing these self-tests, you will not only ensure your safety but will be able to decide which 28-day plan is appropriate for you at this point in your balance journey. It's also important to recognize that the 28-day plans are meant to guide you, and they are designed to allow flexibility, so that you can tailor them for your individual needs. If an exercise feels too easy or too difficult, you can always modify it using the suggestions that we provide, so it works for you.

Just remember to always respect your limits when performing the exercises. It's better to start with an exercise that is too easy and progress from there, especially if you don't feel confident in your abilities yet or feel unsafe doing a particular exercise.

WHEN AND HOW TO PROGRESS TO MORE ADVANCED EXERCISES

Just like when we want to build strength, we need to make sure the weight we are lifting is heavy enough to make progress. Imagine your balance abilities are like a muscle you are trying to train. If it constantly feels "too easy," you will not improve. **When an exercise no longer feels challenging, it's time to increase the challenge**. When you notice the exercise feels "easy," use the modifications we provide with each exercise, to make it more challenging. Likewise, you might be ready to progress to a more advanced version when you notice **significant improvements in your self-assessment**. That's a good sign it is time to step it up!

For example, if the first time you did the tests you were at a high risk of falling, you would have started with the beginner-level 28-day plan. However, if you do the self-assessment again after completing the plan and you are now at a medium risk of falling, it might be time to give the intermediate-level a try so you can keep progressing.

HOW TO ADJUST EXERCISES FOR INCREASED OR DECREASED DIFFICULTY

As mentioned previously, each balance exercise in this book comes with a suggestion on how to make it easier or more challenging. The way to do this is by "playing" with the different balance systems (visual, vestibular, and proprioceptive). When you challenge one or more of these systems, the balance exercises become more difficult.

Here are some examples of how to make balance exercises easier:

- Hold on to a stable object like a chair or countertop.

- Stand on a stable surface like a wooden floor.

- Use a wider base of support.

- Keep your eyes open and focus on something that is not moving.

- Eliminate outside distractions (like loud noises or television programs).

On the other hand, here are some ways to make balance exercises more challenging:

- Close your eyes.
- Add eye or head movement.
- Sit or stand on an uneven surface like a cushion.
- Narrow your base of support.
- Adding a mental task.
- Standing on one leg only.

These modification strategies are also included in each balance exercise description, to remind you of the options you can use. Next, we will discuss how you can integrate balance into your everyday life, and how to make it part of your long-term strategy for well-being.

CHAPTER 10

INTEGRATING BALANCE ACTIVITIES INTO DAILY LIFE FOR LONG-TERM MOBILITY

In addition to following a structured exercise program, it's also possible to improve your balance abilities as part of your daily activities. A study published in the *British Medical Journal* found that integrating balance in everyday activities for older adults resulted in fewer falls after doing so for twelve months (Clemson et al., 2012). That is encouraging news because if you're mindful about it, you can use your daily activities to continue to improve.

Let's go over some examples of how this might look in your everyday life:

1. Take the stairs more often

If you have stairs in your home, that is a good place to start. Make a point to go up and down the stairs throughout the day. Even if you don't have stairs at home, take the stairs instead of the elevator or escalator whenever you can. Every opportunity counts and will benefit you in the long term.

2. Stand in tandem

This foot position is described and illustrated in the balance exercises, if you need a reminder on how to do it. To integrate this into your daily activities, you could take this position when waiting in line at the store, when brushing your teeth, or when talking to someone on the phone.

3. Stand on one leg

This position is also described in the balance exercises, if you need a reminder on how to do it. Just like the tandem stance, it's possible to hold the one-legged stance during everyday activities. You could stand on one leg while something is heating up in the microwave, while you are washing the dishes, or when waiting for the kettle to boil. This stance is more advanced, so make sure you have a sturdy object to hold onto if needed.

4. Mini squats throughout the day

This is an easy technique to integrate throughout the day. For example, when you are reaching for something on the ground, squat, and mindfully pick it up. If you find yourself waiting for something in the kitchen, use the time to do a set of squats. When you are cleaning the house, see if you can do squats instead of simply bending over at the waist as you move around the house and complete your chores. The goal is to integrate balance exercises into your day. It might not seem like you are doing much, but over the course of the day the repetitions will add up.

ONGOING PRACTICE

Congratulations for making it this far, and learning so many new tools for wellness! Starting and establishing a routine is always the most difficult part. As with many things that relate to health, exercise is an ongoing process. Continue to practice the balance exercises you have learned, refer to this book often, and review the essential practices so that you can keep improving your balance for many years to come.

REFERENCES

Borowicz, A., et al. "Assessing Gait and Balance Impairment in Elderly Residents of Nursing Homes." *Journal of Physical Therapy Science*. 28.9 (2016): 2486–2490. https://doi.org/10.1589/jpts.28.2486

Clemson, L., et al. "Integration of Balance and Strength Training into Daily Life Activity to Reduce Rate of Falls in Older People (the LIFE Study): Randomized Parallel Trial." *BMJ* (Clinical Research ed.). 345 (2012): e4547. https://doi.org/10.1136/bmj.e4547

Erickson, K. I., et al. "Exercise Training Increases Size of Hippocampus and Improves Memory." *Proceedings of the National Academy of Sciences of the United States of America*. 108.7 (2011): 3017–3022. https://doi.org/10.1073/pnas.1015950108

Izquierdo, M., et al. "International Exercise Recommendations in Older Adults: Expert Consensus Guidelines." *The Journal of Nutrition, Health & Aging*. 25.7 (2021): 824–853. https://doi.org/10.1007/s12603-021-1665-8

Madhushri, P., et al. "A Health Tool Suite for Mobility Assessment." *Inf.*, 7.47 (2016).

Myers, A. M., et al. "Discriminative and Evaluative Properties of the Activities-Specific Balance Confidence (ABC) Scale." *The Journal of Gerontology: Series A, Biological Sciences and Medical Sciences*. 53.4 (1998): M287–M294. https://doi.org/10.1093/gerona/53a.4.m287

National Institute on Aging. "Falls and Falls Prevention: Older Adults and Balance Problems."

National Institute on Aging. "10 Myths About Aging."

O'Sullivan, S. B., Schmitz, T. J., & Fulk, G. D. *Physical Rehabilitation*, 6th edition.

Peterka R. J. "Sensory Integration for Human Balance Control." *Handbook of Clinical Neurology*. 159 (2018): 27–42. https://doi.org/10.1016/B978-0-444-63916-5.00002-1

Phelan, E. A., Mahoney, J. E., Voit, J. C., & Stevens, J. A. "Assessment and Management of Fall Risk in Primary Care Settings." *The Medical Clinics of North America*. 99.2 (2015), 281–293. https://doi.org/10.1016/j.mcna.2014.11.004

Rivera-Torres, S., Fahey, T. D., & Rivera, M. A. "Adherence to Exercise Programs in Older Adults: Informative Report." *Gerontology & Geriatric Medicine*. 5 (2019). https://doi.org/10.1177/2333721418823604

Saftari, L. N., & Kwon, O. S. "Aging Vision and Falls: A Review." *Journal of Physiological Anthropology*. 37.1 (2018): 11. https://doi.org/10.1186/s40101-018-0170-1

Sherrington, C., et al. "Exercise for Preventing Falls in Older People Living in the Community." *The Cochrane Database of Systematic Reviews*. 1.1 (2019): CD012424. https://doi.org/10.1002/14651858.CD012424.pub2

Stanghelle, B., et al. "Effects of a Resistance and Balance Exercise Programme on Physical Fitness, Health-Related Quality of Life and Fear of Falling in Older Women with Osteoporosis and Vertebral Fracture: A Randomized Controlled Trial." *Osteoporosis International*. 31.6 (2020): 1069–1078. https://doi.org/10.1007/s00198-019-05256-4

Thomas, E., et al. "Physical Activity Programs for Balance and Fall Prevention in Elderly: A Systematic Review." *Medicine*. 98.27 (2019): e16218. https://doi.org/10.1097/MD.0000000000016218

BONUS THANK YOU

Thank you for choosing **Fall Prevention Balance Exercises for Seniors**. We hope this book has provided you with the guidance and inspiration needed to embark on your fitness journey. Your commitment to improving your health and well-being is truly commendable.

Remember, every small step you take brings you closer to a healthier, happier you. Keep going, and stay motivated!

Don't forget to claim your bonus. Go to your internet browser and type in **www.getmovefit.com/balance** to register for the unlimited and free portal access. There are no hidden extra costs, this is completely free with the purchase of this book.

SCAN ME

The PIN code to unlock your bonus is **13597**

WE ARE HERE TO HELP!

Contact us at **support@getmovefit.com** and we will reply within 2 business days.

These bonuses are **FREE** and designed to **help you achieve your goals**.

With gratitude,
Linette Cunley

www.ingramcontent.com/pod-product-compliance
Lightning Source LLC
Chambersburg PA
CBHW080000280326
41935CB00013B/1701